Ethics in Sports Medicine

Editor

STEPHEN R. THOMPSON

CLINICS IN SPORTS MEDICINE

www.sportsmed.theclinics.com

Consulting Editor
MARK D. MILLER

April 2016 • Volume 35 • Number 2

ELSEVIER

1600 John F. Kennedy Boulevard ● Suite 1800 ● Philadelphia, Pennsylvania, 19103-2899

http://www.theclinics.com

CLINICS IN SPORTS MEDICINE Volume 35, Number 2

April 2016 ISSN 0278-5919, ISBN 13: 978-0-323-41771-6

Editor: Jennifer Flynn-Briggs
Developmental Editor: Donald Mumford

Clinics in Sports Medicine (ISSN 0278-5919) is published quarterly by Elsevier Inc., 360 Park Avenue South, New York, NY 10010-1710. Months of issue are January, April, July, and October. Business and Editorial Offices: 1600 John F. Kennedy Blvd., Ste. 1800, Philadelphia, PA 19103-2899. Customer Service Office: 3251 Riverport Lane, Maryland Heights, MO 63043. Periodicals postage paid at New York, NY and additional mailing offices. Subscription prices are $340.00 per year (US individuals), $597.00 per year (US institutions), $100.00 per year (US students), $385.00 per year (Canadian individuals), $737.00 per year (Canadian institutions), $235.00 (Canadian students), $470.00 per year (foreign individuals), $737.00 per year (foreign institutions), and $235.00 per year (foreign students). Foreign air speed delivery is included in all *Clinics* subscription prices. All prices are subject to change without notice. **POSTMASTER:** Send address changes to *Clinics in Sports Medicine*, Elsevier Health Sciences Division, Subscription Customer Service, 3251 Riverport Lane, Maryland Heights, MO 63043. Customer Service (orders, claims, online, change of address): Elsevier Health Sciences Division, Subscription Customer Service, 3251 Riverport Lane, Maryland Heights, MO 63043. **Tel: 1-800-654-2452 (U.S. and Canada); 314-447-8871 (outside U.S. and Canada). Fax: 314-447-8029. E-mail: journalscustomerservice-usa@elsevier.com (for print support); journalsonlinesupport-usa@elsevier.com (for online support)**.

Reprints. For copies of 100 or more of articles in this publication, please contact the Commercial Reprints Department, Elsevier Inc., 360 Park Avenue South, New York, NY 10010-1710. Tel.: 212-633-3874; Fax: 212-633-3820; E-mail: reprints@elsevier.com.

Clinics in Sports Medicine is covered in *MEDLINE/PubMed (Index Medicus) Current Contents/Clinical Medicine, Excerpta Medica,* and *ISI/Biomed.*

Contributors

CONSULTING EDITOR

MARK D. MILLER, MD
S. Ward Casscells Professor, Head, Division of Sports Medicine, Department of Orthopaedic Surgery, University of Virginia, Charlottesville, Virginia; Team Physician, James Madison University, Harrisonburg, Virginia

EDITOR

STEPHEN R. THOMPSON, MD, MEd, FRCSC
Cooperating Associate Professor of Sports Medicine, The University of Maine; Medical Director, EMMC Sports Health, Eastern Maine Medical Center, Bangor, Maine

AUTHORS

LYNLEY ANDERSON, MSc, PhD
Division of Health Sciences, University of Otago, Dunedin, New Zealand

B. SONNY BAL, MD, JD, MBA
Department of Orthopedic Surgery, University of Missouri, Columbia, Missouri

ANDREW BLOODWORTH, BSc, PhD
Lecturer in Philosophy and Ethics of Healthcare, College of Human and Health Sciences, Swansea University, Swansea, United Kingdom

LAWRENCE H. BRENNER, JD
Department of Orthopaedics and Rehabilitation, Yale University, New Haven, Connecticut

RAFF CALITRI, BSc (Hons), MSc, PhD
Research Fellow, Psychology Applied to Health, University of Exeter Medical School, Exeter, United Kingdom

SILVIA CAMPORESI, PhD, PhD
Department of Social Science, Health and Medicine, King's College London, London, United Kingdom

BRIAN M. DEVITT, MD, FRSC
Director of Research, Consultant Orthopaedic Surgeon, OrthoSport Victoria, Melbourne, Victoria, Australia

DIONNE L. KOLLER, JD, MA
Associate Professor of Law and Director, Center for Sport and the Law, University of Baltimore School of Law, Baltimore, Maryland

DOMINIC MALCOLM, BA, MA, PhD
Reader in Sociology of Sport, School of Sport, Exercise and Health Sciences, Loughborough University, Leicestershire, United Kingdom

MATTHEW J. MATAVA, MD
Professor and Chief of Sports Medicine, Department of Orthopedic Surgery, Washington University, St Louis, Missouri

MICHAEL J. McNAMEE, BA, MA, MA, PhD
Professor of Applied Ethics, College of Engineering, Swansea University, Swansea, United Kingdom

BRADLEY PARTRIDGE, BSc, PhD
Faculty of Health and Behavioural Sciences, The University of Queensland, St Lucia, Queensland, Australia

CAROLINE POMA, BA
University of North Carolina School of Law, Chapel Hill, North Carolina; University of Virginia, Charlottesville, Virginia

BRUCE REIDER, MD
Department of Orthopaedics and Rehabilitation Medicine, The University of Chicago Medicine, Chicago, Illinois

SETH L. SHERMAN, MD
Department of Orthopedic Surgery, University of Missouri, Columbia, Missouri

BRADLEY SPENCE, BA
University of Missouri School of Medicine, Columbia, Missouri

ROBERT J. STEWART, MD
Department of Orthopaedics and Rehabilitation Medicine, The University of Chicago Medicine, Chicago, Illinois

JACINTA OON AI TAN, MBBS, MA, MRCPsych, DPhil, MSc
Clinical Associate Professor of Psychiatry, Institute of Life Sciences 2, College of Medicine, Swansea University, Swansea, United Kingdom

ANDREW M. TUCKER, MD
Medical Director, Medstar Union Memorial Sports Medicine, Baltimore, Maryland

Contents

> In sports medicine, the practice of ethics presents many unique challenges because of the unusual clinical environment of caring for players within the context of a team whose primary goal is to win. Ethical issues frequently arise because a doctor-patient-team triad often replaces the traditional doctor-patient relationship. Conflict may exist when the team's priority clashes with or even replaces the doctor's obligation to player well-being. Customary ethical norms that govern most forms of clinical practice, such as autonomy and confidentiality, are not easily translated to sports medicine. Ethical principles and examples of how they relate to sports medicine are discussed.

> This article synthesizes existing literature to provide a summary of the ethical issues concerning patient confidentiality in sport. It outlines the medical principle of confidentiality and identifies cross-cultural ethicolegal variations that shape its implementation. Clinicians' multiple obligations, physical environments, and practice and policy contexts are discussed, and research detailing experiences of maintaining patient confidentiality in sport is reviewed. Policy recommendations for enhancing compliance with this ethical principle are summarized. It is argued that the context of sport exacerbates pressures on clinicians to break patient confidentiality, breaches occur regularly, and interventions are required to enhance ethical compliance in sports medicine.

> Conflict of interest is common in the practice of medicine, and likely more so in the practice of sports medicine at the highest levels of competition. Two areas where conflict of interest frequently manifest in sports medicine are confidentiality and clinical decision making. Confidentiality can be challenging by the team physician's dual responsibilities to the player-patient and the team. Clinical decision making, traditionally associated with a patient's long term health interests, can be complicated by short term interests rooted in pursuit of winning. These issues are reviewed, hopefully

This article provides an overview of commonly used analgesics in athletes and the ethical implications of their use in athletic settings. Given the highly competitive nature of modern-day sports and the economic impact of athletic performance at elite levels, athletes feel more compelled than ever to play with injury, which has led to the widespread use of a variety of analgesic agents. An ethical dilemma often ensues for team physicians who must balance the medical implications of these drugs with pressure from players, coaches, and management. The most commonly used agents and their ethical and rational use are discussed.

The recognition of sports medicine and promulgation of practice guidelines for team physicians will push general medical malpractice standards to evolve into a more specialized standard of care for those who practice in this area. To the extent that practicing medicine in the sports context involves calculations that do not arise in typical medical practice, the sports medicine community can help elucidate those issues and create appropriate guidelines that can serve to inform athlete–patients and educate courts. Doing so will help best set the terms by which those who practice sports medicine are judged.

Despite considerable scientific dispute regarding the science of concussion, there has been a proliferation of position statements and professional guidelines published on sports concussion management over the last 15 years. A number of ethical and clinical problems associated with concussion management protocols remain concerning, (i) diagnosis and management; (ii) conflicts of interest and coercion; (iii) same day return to play; and (iv) reporting, auditing and confidentiality. These issues are critically discussed in the light of recent Consensus Statements. It is argued that the use of independent match day doctors may ameliorate some of these concerns.

There is public discussion and debate about the role of the team physician in professional sports. There is uncertainty over whether a separate legal standard of care should apply when treating professional athletes. This article advocates a single standard of care for all patients. This article also proposes that it would be useful for team physicians to develop a consensus that there should be a health policy for professional athletes.

This health policy should aspire to assert that professional athletes can complete their career, while minimizing the risk of cognitive or physical injuries that affect later quality of life.

Jacinta Oon Ai Tan, Raff Calitri, Andrew Bloodworth, and Michael J. McNamee

Eating disorders and disordered eating are more common in high performance sports than the general population, and particularly so in high performance aesthetic sports. This paper presents some of the conceptual difficulties in understanding and diagnosing eating disorders in high performance gymnasts. It presents qualitative and quantitative data from a study designed to ascertain the pattern of eating disorder symptoms, depressive symptoms and levels of self-esteem among national and international level gymnasts from the UK in the gymnastic disciplines of sport acrobatics, tumbling, and rhythmic gymnastics.

Silvia Camporesi

The International Association for Athletics Federations (IAAF) has been granted 2 years to submit further evidence showing a correlation between higher levels of testosterone and a competitive advantage. This article first presents the case of Caster Semenya, which triggered the drafting by IAAF of the regulations on eligibility of female athletes to compete in the female category in 2011. Then the IAAF regulations are critically analyzed from a scientific and ethical point of view. Finally, the Court of Arbitration for Sport decision to suspend the regulations pending further evidence provided by IAAF, and what this means for the future of sports, is discussed.

Robert J. Stewart and Bruce Reider

This article explores the background and foundations of ethics in research. Some important documents and codes are mentioned, such as The Belmont Report and the International Council for Harmonisation. Some influential historical events involving research ethics are recounted. The article provides a detailed discussion of the Declaration of Helsinki, which is considered the international standard for guidelines in medical research ethics. The most salient features of the Declaration are described and related to orthopaedic surgery and sports medicine. Some of the most controversial aspects of the Declaration are discussed, which helps examine contentious areas of research in sports medicine.

CLINICS IN SPORTS MEDICINE

THE CLINICS ARE AVAILABLE ONLINE!
Access your subscription at:
www.theclinics.com

Foreword

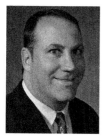

Mark D. Miller, MD
Consulting Editor

Ethics in sports medicine is very much a gray area. There are limited resources to consult, and, often, no "correct" answers. Nevertheless, this is a fundamental part of being a team physician. Dr Stephen Thompson has taken on the challenge of providing some much needed guidance on ethical issues in this issue of *Clinics in Sports Medicine*. Steve has summarized this issue in a well-written preface, so there is no need to rehash that here. Suffice it to say that there are some important pearls here that we all need to learn. Thank-you, Dr Thompson, and all the authors, for an excellent issue of *Clinics in Sports Medicine*.

Mark D. Miller, MD
Department of Orthopaedic Surgery
University of Virginia

James Madison University
400 Ray C. Hunt Drive, Suite 330
Charlottesville, VA 22908, USA

E-mail address:
mdm3p@virginia.edu

Clin Sports Med 35 (2016) ix
http://dx.doi.org/10.1016/j.csm.2015.11.002
0278-5919/16/$ – see front matter © 2016 Published by Elsevier Inc.

sportsmed.theclinics.com

Preface

Ethics and the Sports Medicine Physician

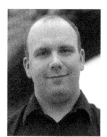

Stephen R. Thompson, MD, MEd, FRCSC
Editor

It is clear that whoever is a physician must be altogether a philosopher.

— *Galen*

The practice of sports medicine enables many unique opportunities to the physician but also results in several unique challenges. One particular challenge is practicing in an ethical fashion. There are multiple scenarios that occur in the office, in the training room, and on the field that result in ethical dilemmas. Navigating these issues is not always easy, and, often, there is no clear direction to take.

The purpose of this issue is to provide the basic ethical framework to the sports medicine physician to enable them to tackle these challenges head on. We have been fortunate to have contributions from a wide array of authors. Several are physicians who practice at the highest levels of professional sports, while others are philosophers, ethicists, and attorneys.

To begin, Dr Devit lays the groundwork in his article on "Fundamental Ethical Principles in Sports Medicine." Next, Dr Malcolm provides guidance on how to handle patient confidentiality in a sports medicine practice in his article on "Confidentiality in Sports Medicine." Invariably, caring for athletes results in a conflict of interest owing to the "patient-physician-team" triad. Dr Tucker leans on his many years of professional team medical coverage on how to handle these conflicts in his article on "Conflicts of Interest in Sports Medicine."

Similarly, within the professional environment, the physician can experience the unique challenges associated with analgesic use to mask pain and improve performance. Dr Matava, also a professional team physician, outlines the different regulations and best practices in his article, "Ethical Considerations for Analgesic Use in Sports Medicine."

Clin Sports Med 35 (2016) xi–xii
http://dx.doi.org/10.1016/j.csm.2015.11.001
0278-5919/16/$ – see front matter © 2016 Published by Elsevier Inc.

sportsmed.theclinics.com

Ethics and the law often coexist, and Professor Koller provides a comprehensive review of important ethical and legal aspects as they relate to the practice of sports medicine in her article, "Team Physicians, Sports Medicine, and the Law: An Update." Following this, Professor McNamee, Professor Partridge, and Professor Anderson detail their thinking of ethics surrounding concussion care in their very seminal article, "Concussion Ethics and Sports Medicine."

Closely related to this are issues of standards of care in professional athletes who are often willing to have "substandard" care for better short-term performance but to the detriment of their long-term health. Drs Poma, Sherman, Spence, Brenner, and Bal use their combined medical and legal experience to propose a series of guidelines to define a standard of care in their article, "Rethinking the Standard of Care in Treating Professional Athletes."

Finally, there is a set of very unique ethical issues within sports medicine that warrants further discussion. Drs Tan, Calitri, Bloodworth, and McNamee discuss the ethics surrounding eating disorders in gymnasts in their article, "Understanding Eating Disorders in Elite Gymnastics: Ethical and Conceptual Challenges." Professor Camporesi then provides a thought provoking article on the ethics of concussion management in her article, "Ethics of Regulating Competition for Women with Hyperandrogenism." Last, we would never advance without research into our practice, and Drs Steward and Reider detail the important ethical principles of research in the article, "The Ethics of Sports Medicine Research."

I am indebted to this outstanding multidisciplinary group of individuals, who have provided insightful and clear discussion on this frequently encountered but rarely taught subject. As Galen wrote, "...that the best physician is also a philosopher."

Stephen R. Thompson, MD, MEd, FRCSC
The University of Maine
Eastern Maine Medical Center
925 Union Street, Suite 3
Bangor, ME 04401, USA

E-mail address:
theskip@gmail.com

Fundamental Ethical Principles in Sports Medicine

Brian M. Devitt, MD, FRSC

KEYWORDS

- Ethics • Sports medicine • Deontology • Utilitarianism • Autonomy
- Virtuous practice

KEY POINTS

- The practice of ethics in sports medicine is challenging because a doctor-patient-team triad often replaces the traditional doctor-patient relationship.
- For many ethical dilemmas, there are no right answers, but knowledge of the principles and exposure to the practice of ethics are helpful in making sound decisions.
- The value of an athlete is never merely instrumental, and athletes should be regarded as ends in themselves, not means.
- Medical personnel may have passion for a sport but must show dispassion in the execution of their medical duties and always demonstrate professional conduct.
- Player autonomy is crucial in sports medicine: "do not abdicate your responsibility to the individual player."

INTRODUCTION

Ethics at its simplest is the study of what makes a particular action in a particular circumstance the right thing to do. In sports medicine, the practice of ethics presents many unique challenges because of the unusual clinical environment of caring for players within the context of a team whose primary goal is to win.[1] Consequently, the traditional doctor-patient relationship is often distorted or absent. A doctor-patient-team triad frequently exists, which creates a scenario in which the team's priority can conflict with or even supplant the doctor's primary obligation to player well-being.[2] As such, the customary ethical norms that govern most forms of clinical practice, such as patient confidentiality and autonomy, are not easily translated into sports medicine.

Disclosure Statement: The author has nothing to disclose.
OrthoSport Victoria, Level 5 Epworth Hospital, 89 Bridge Road, Melbourne, Victoria 3121, Australia
E-mail address: bdevitt@hotmail.com

Clin Sports Med 35 (2016) 195–204
http://dx.doi.org/10.1016/j.csm.2015.10.004
sportsmed.theclinics.com

Sports doctors are frequently under intense pressure to keep athletes on the field of play and improve performance. This burden, whether implicit or explicit, from management, coaches, trainers, and agents, may compel medical personnel to opt for short-term solutions to injury rather than consider the long-term sequelae of such decisions.[3] A variety of ethical dilemmas may be encountered, and for many of these dilemmas, there are no unique right answers. Several ethical approaches have been proposed to deal with the wide range of complex and challenging ethical problems faced in Medicine; these may be broadly classified into the following areas:

Deontology
Utilitarianism
Principles Approach
Virtuous Practice

No single approach provides the solution to every ethical issue, and quite often these ethical standpoints conflict with each other. A detailed understanding of each of these ethical philosophies is probably not necessary in most cases. However, an awareness of the core concepts is extremely useful in sports medicine to provide a framework for decision-making and ethical practice.

In this article, these ethical approaches and how they relate to sports medicine are discussed. In doing so, a comparison is made between some of the more contrasting ethical standpoints. Also, several clinical vignettes are included to illustrate certain ethical dilemmas. To conclude, a list of guidelines has been drawn up to offer some support to doctors facing an ethical quandary. The most important guideline is "do not abdicate your responsibility to the individual player."

SPORT AND THE HISTORY OF ETHICS IN SPORTS MEDICINE

Sport plays an integral role in society and naturally serves as a vehicle for education, health, leadership, and fair play. One of the core principles of sport is fairness, which can be used as a metaphor for behavior in everyday life. The true ethos of sport is epitomized in an informal motto of the Olympic games: "The most important thing is not to win but to take part!" However, whether this ethos is adhered to depends on how the sport is managed, taught, and practiced.

Sport has clearly become a global enterprise as well as a recreation for billions.[4] Nowadays, athletes can demand lucrative sponsorship contracts and appearance fees. Recently, Floyd Mayweather topped the Forbes list of the highest paid athletes in sport, earning $US300 million in a single year, more than double the previous high for an athlete.[5] As the commercialization of sport increases, the value of victory in monetary terms has never been greater. Accordingly, the pressure on athletes to win has increased considerably as have the demands on sports-medicine doctors to facilitate this success by whatever means.

There has long been an adversarial relationship between sporting performance and patient welfare, which stretches back to early Greek and Roman civilization. Aelius Galenus, regarded as one of the forefathers of sports medicine, served as a physician to the gladiators in Pergamum in AD 157. He argued vehemently against the immoderate lifestyle of athletes and their obsession with victory, which he believed was unhealthy and potentially dangerous behavior.[6] He saw himself as both a physician and a philosopher, and he believed the 2 were integrally linked, which he outlined in a small treatise he wrote called, "That the Best Physician Is Also a Philosopher."[7] His theories have dominated and influenced Western medical science for well over a millennium.

DEONTOLOGY (GREEK: DEON = DUTY)

Patients must be able to trust doctors with their lives and health. To justify that trust, doctors must show respect for human life and ensure their practice meets the standards expected by the public and medical governing bodies.[8] Deontology is known as duty-based ethics. This approach, the best-known proponent of which was the philosopher Immanuel Kant (1724–1804), is based on the premise of what distinguishes mankind from other animals is their ability to reason and to use this reason to determine what actions are right.[9,10] It follows that all humans have universal rational duties to one another and, most importantly, must respect one another's humanity. Kant maintained that all humans must be seen as inherently worthy of respect and dignity. Moreover, he contended that all morality must stem from such duties. Put simply, the primary tenet of this ethical principle is to do the right thing because it is the right thing to do.

Kant determined that there were certain general obligations to consider when deciding on an action, which he referred to as the categorical imperatives. The first categorical imperative instructs to "act only by that maxim by which you can, at the same time, will that it be a universal law." In other words, when considering what you should do in a certain situation, you must ask yourself "would it be acceptable if everyone took this type of action?"

CLINICAL VIGNETTE: CONCUSSION

There are numerous examples of how this imperative may be applied in a sporting context. Consider the topical example of managing a player with a concussion: Therefore, if one day it would be beneficial to let your star athlete play on in a game with concussion, you should ask yourself, "would it be acceptable if every player with concussion played on?" Clearly the answer is no, because to do so would put the athletes under your care at an unacceptable risk and be morally wrong.

Players as Ends Not Means

The second categorical imperative states: "So act as to treat humanity, whether in your own person or in that of any other, in every case as an end in itself, never as a means only." This principle does not always fit easily with the ethos of many sports teams. In changing rooms before games, players are often told to "put your body on the line" for the cause of the team. Although this saying is intended to promote selflessness not recklessness, it does highlight that the professional obligations of the medical staff are not always aligned with the motivations of the management and coaching staff. The success of the team must never supersede the welfare of individual players. Of course, individual players may be integral to the success of the team, but they must always be treated with all the respect due to a person. Therefore, the value of a person is never merely instrumental, and players should be regarded as ends in themselves, not means.

Although the principle of duty-based ethics is appealing, applying it in the context of a sporting environment is not always so straightforward. One of the core teachings of deontology is that people have a duty to do the right thing, regardless of the good or bad consequences that may be produced.[10] As a result, an action cannot be justified by showing that it produced good consequences, or condemned if it produces bad consequences, which is why it is sometimes called non-Consequentialist. This approach is in stark contrast to principles of utilitarianism, which promote Consequentialism.

UTILITARIANISM

"There is no 'I' in team"

This cliché is a frequent exhortation in prematch talks. It advocates the concept of putting the team before the individual, which forms the basis of utilitarianism. As a system of ethics, utilitarianism directs that the rightness or wrongness of an action should be judged by its consequences. The goal of utilitarian ethics is to promote the greatest happiness for the greatest number of individuals, which in a sporting context represents the team. To those solely focused on the success of the team alone, this approach is attractive because it seems to provide an empirical solution to ethical dilemmas. It provides a method of weighing up the potential benefits and harms of an action, so that a balanced judgment can be made on the proportionate benefit that can be achieved. The greater the excess of benefit over potential or actual harm, then the more likely it is that the action can be justified. In essence, sporting organizations want to do what is the right for the good of the sporting organization.

However, the primary role of the team doctor is not simply to ensure the success of the team or the sporting organization. The problem with this approach is that it denigrates the interests of individual players in favor of the team's interest. Put another way, certain parties may justify jeopardizing the welfare of one or more players in the pursuit of success for the team. This stance must never be that of the team doctor.

> **CLINICAL VIGNETTE: THE TOURING TEAM**
>
> *Nevertheless, there are certain situations in a team environment in which a utilitarian approach is appropriate. Consider the example of dealing with an injured player while on tour: The doctor is charged with the responsibility of ensuring the well-being of the entire player group. If the time and resources necessary to treat and rehabilitate an individual player and allow them to remain on tour are so demanding as to potentially have a negative impact on the medical services available for the rest of the group, a decision might be made to send the player home for further treatment.*

Consequentialism Versus Non-Consequentialism

It is obvious that utilitarianism and deontology offer rather contrasting ethical standpoints on what are the right actions to take. Therefore, how does one decide which approach to adopt? Consequentialists start by considering what a good outcome is and identify right actions as the ones that produce the maximum of those good outcomes.[11] However, one of the arguments to favor a duty-based rather than consequence-based approach is that, despite a person's best efforts, the future is uncertain and cannot be controlled. Therefore, a person should be praised or blamed for the actions within their control, and that includes willing and not achieving.

Then again, the problem with deontology is that it yields only absolutes. Actions are considered right or wrong with no allowances for gray areas. By strictly adhering to the rigid moral laws, there is no room for even a white lie or gamesmanship, for example, in comforting a player coming off the field or giving a slightly overoptimistic prognosis to improve a player's morale. Moral dilemmas are created when duties come in conflict, and there is no mechanism for solving them. With Utilitarianism, if a set of alternatives has the same expected utility, they are all equally good. The problem here, though, is that predicting future outcomes is a very inexact science.

PRINCIPLES ETHICS

Principles ethics is one of the most well-known and perhaps the most useful ethical approaches in practical terms. Generally regarded as the most appropriate method for approaching medical ethical dilemmas, it is based on the four pillars of autonomy, beneficence, nonmaleficence, and justice.[2]

Autonomy

Respect for a patient's autonomy is considered a fundamental ethical principle. Autonomy denotes the capacity of a rational individual to make an informed, uncoerced decision. This belief is central to the premise of the concept of informed consent. The principle of confidentiality is also essential in patient autonomy. A player must give informed consent for confidential information to be divulged to the management team.

This area is of particular relevance to sports medicine personnel when dealing with an injured player who is faced with a treatment choice. The sports doctor must ensure the player not only understands the injury but also understands the risks and benefits of all possible treatment options, and the future prognosis.

Clinical Vignette: Meniscal Injury in Season

The commonly used clinical example to illustrate this dilemma is the young, professional football player who tears his medial meniscus midway through the season. The tear is reparable but the player is faced with two choices: he can undergo an arthroscopic meniscectomy and return to play relatively quickly or undergo a meniscal repair and be out for the rest of the season. The result of each procedure may have short-term and long-term consequences. In the short term, the player who chooses to have the meniscectomy may return to play more quickly, whereas the player who opts for a meniscal repair faces a longer period of rehabilitation and will miss more game time. In the long term, the player who opts for a meniscectomy substantially increases his chances of developing degenerative arthritis in his knee in the future, whereas the player who chooses a meniscal repair has the chance of pain-free function in the longer term and probable avoidance of articular degeneration.[12,13]

Informed consent in clinical sports medicine takes on a greater level of importance than in normal clinical circumstance because of all the added pressures and influences. The consequences of the player's decision extend further than his own well-being and have an effect on his team and coach. The consent process may be compromised by the fact that different parties in the triad of relationships may have different values and priorities, and therefore, might choose different options.[6] This case highlights several important questions. In what ways can the sports-medicine doctor recognize that the team has a legitimate stake in the outcome and yet remain loyal to the player? Should the physician seek consensus with all the parties involved?[2] Although these are all very relevant and salient questions, the answer is simple. The primary obligation of the sports-medicine doctor is to the patient. Patient autonomy always supplants the doctor's partiality.[6] Although the paymaster in professional sport is the team, sports-medicine doctors cannot abdicate their responsibility to the individual player. The burden of obligation to the team should be removed from the team doctor, thereby rejecting the utilitarian doctrine. It is the player's right to determine what is in his best interest. Nonetheless, as a patient advocate, the doctor must be acutely aware that the player is often under external pressure from teammates, coaches, and agents as well as internal drives and goals that may influence treatment decisions.[2] In fact, there is a responsibility of the team doctor to tease out the extent of influence on a player to make a certain decision in the process of informed consent.[3]

The International Federation of Sports Medicine guidelines also prove useful in such a scenario: "Never impose your authority in a way that impinges on the individual right of the athlete to make his/her own decisions" and "A basic ethical principle in healthcare is that of respect for autonomy. An essential component of autonomy is knowledge. Failure to obtain informed consent is to undermine the athlete's autonomy."[14]

Beneficence

The second principle, beneficence, directs that health care professionals should aim to "do good" and promote the interest of their patients. It is one of the core values of health care ethics and is important in elucidating the nature and goals of medicine as a social practice. Edmund Pelligrino[15] argues that beneficence is the only fundamental principle of medical ethics, that healing should be the sole purpose of medicine, and that endeavors like cosmetic surgery and contraception fall beyond its remit.

The very nature of sport is that it can occasionally harm and involves various degrees of risk, and thus, raises the question of how of a doctor can stand by idly and watch this happen without intervening. This question brings us back to the adversarial relationship between participation in sport and personal welfare. Players participate in sport of their own volition and need to be aware of the inherent risks they face. The principal motivation of the sports-medicine doctor is one of beneficence, and the primary aim is to do good for the patient by treating any injuries that may occur and prevent any further harm.

Nonmaleficence: Primum Non Nocere (First, Do No Harm)

The third principle requires that doctors should do no harm. Conflicts are evident between beneficence and nonmaleficence in almost any clinical situation. The dichotomy between the two principles is the foundation for risk/benefit analysis. The principles of beneficence and nonmaleficence should be considered together and aim at producing an excess of benefit over harm, in keeping with traditional Hippocratic moral obligation.[16] The obligation to provide net benefit to patients requires that there is a clear or as clear as possible discernment of risk profiles when an assessment of harm and benefit is made.

Beneficence Versus Nonmaleficence

A difficult situation arises when players adopt a somewhat cavalier approach to their own careers and, more importantly, welfare. In such a scenario, the short-term glory a player stands to gain by playing with injury more than compensates for the risk of long-term disability. Players enter into sport knowing that injury and harm are an occupational hazard. However, the medical team must try their best to limit that risk or, at the very least, prevent further harm to the player when injured. There is no obligation on players to choose the recommended treatment plan put forward by the doctor, but at the very least they need to be aware of the risks and consequences of their decisions. Equally, medical staff must respect a player's decision even if it is contrary to their own opinion. In such circumstances, the sporting governing body has an important overseeing role to provide guidelines on controversial treatment.

CLINICAL VIGNETTE: I NEED A SHOT, DOC!

The team doctor is approached by the coach at half-time asking him to give his star player a shot of local anesthetic into his knee to allow him finish out the game.

The administration of local anesthetic to allow a player to return to participation is a controversial issue and one that poses an import ethical dilemma. Although considered by some to be a performance-enhancing drug, the World Anti-Doping Agency does not list local anesthetic as a prohibited medication.[17] In professional sport, the use of local anesthetic has been shown to permit athletes to return more quickly to participation and, when administered for minor injuries, has been found to be relatively safe.[18,19] However, in certain cases, performance is not enhanced and injuries can be worsened, leading to long-term disability.[19] In most circumstances, when faced with such a scenario, the doctor and player have a choice: accept the benefit of the short-term gain to play on but run the risk of further worsening an injury; or choose not to play on, permitting a more thorough assessment of the injury, but potentially lose out on an opportunity for sporting success. However, this is not the case in rugby. World Rugby, the sport's governing body, dictates that, "A player may not receive local anaesthetics on Match Day unless it is for the suturing of bleeding wounds or for dental treatment administered by an appropriately qualified medical or dental practitioner."[20]

In this circumstance, the position of the doctor is simpler, and the ethical quandary has been removed by virtue of the regulation. If the doctor were to acquiesce to the coach's request, it would not only put the player at risk of potential injury but also expose them to sanction by both the sporting regulatory authority and possibly the doctor's professional body. Admittedly, this type of regulation does not remove the frustration suffered by the player or diminish the doctor's desire to help the patient, but it is protective for both parties.

Justice

The fourth principle is justice. Health care professionals should act fairly when the interests of different individuals or groups are in competition. The obligations of justice may be divided into three categories: fair distribution of scant resources (distributive justice), respect for people's rights (rights-based justice), and respect for morally acceptable laws (legal justice).[16] Distributive justice is relevant to sports medicine in the context of limited resources. If resources are scarce, they should be distributed equally based on need and not on the basis of star talent.

As regards rights-based justice, the team doctor should respect each individual's right to treatment, should they require it. Failure to act because of personal bias or contrary beliefs would be unjust. Finally, the principle of legal justice holds that the team doctor must not willfully cause bodily harm to a player or do anything in contravention of morally acceptable laws.

VIRTUE ETHICS

Although the principle approach is very useful in most moral dilemmas in medicine, it does have limitations. When there are conflicting principles, it is not always easy to decide which principle should dominate. The principle's framework does not take into account the emotional element of human experience. Another approach to bear in mind is the concept of virtue ethics, which emphasizes the character of the practitioner, or moral agent, as the key element of ethical thinking. This approach holds that morality stems from the identity or character of the individual, rather than being a reflection of the actions of the individual.

Therefore, what specific virtues are morally praiseworthy, and how do they relate to the practice of sports medicine? Much of the teaching on virtue ethics is derived from the ancient Greek philosophers. Aristotle believed that a virtue lay at the center point between two divergent vices and referred to it as "the mean by reference to two vices: the one of excess and the other of deficiency." Courage, for example, lies between foolhardiness and cowardice. Compassion lies between callousness and indulgence.[21] Plato believed in the four cardinal virtues: wisdom, justice, fortitude, and temperance.[22] Beauchamp and Childress[23] considered there to be five virtues, which were applicable to the medical practitioner: trustworthiness, integrity, discernment, compassion, and conscientiousness. Nevertheless, there is no comprehensive list of virtues. The Scottish philosopher, MacIntyre,[24] believed that any account of the virtues must indeed be generated out of the community in which those virtues are to be practiced.

His approach also seeks to demonstrate that good judgment emanates from good character. The application of virtue ethics to the sports medicine field may have some advantages over the principles approach. It considers the motivation of the team doctor (agent) to be of crucial importance. Ethical decision-making hinges on the characteristic virtuous disposition of the team doctor, who typically wants to behave well and in the best interest of the player. As there are no strict rules to be obeyed, it permits the adaptation of choices to the particulars of a situation and the people involved. This flexibility promotes creative thinking and problem solving to deal with complex dilemmas. In applying virtue ethics, it is important to be aware that tragic dilemmas can rarely be resolved to the complete satisfaction of all parties and may leave some remainder of pain and regret.[21] Aristotle also believed the virtues could be taught and improved with practice.[21]

Discussion

Sport is conducted in a highly charged and emotional environment. Medical personnel who engage in sports medicine frequently become involved in sport because they too are passionate about the sport. However, this passion may conflict with their ability to be dispassionate about the outcome of the game, especially when dealing with injured players. It is important to accept that medical personnel, as individuals, are not infallible, and medical decisions may be influenced by the appeal of status, admiration, and gratitude.[2] Such behavior is self-gratifying, compromises judgment, and detracts from the primary responsibility of the medical team, which is to preserve player welfare. In this article, a list of guidelines has been drawn up to offer some support to doctors facing an ethical quandary (**Box 1**).

"Fail to prepare, prepare to fail"

Sports medical personnel must remember at all times the importance of ethical medical practice and professional conduct. Exposure to ethical dilemmas and the resultant practice one gets from dealing with these situations can be very helpful in making sound and considered ethical decisions. Indeed, the teaching of ethics should form an important part of the training programs in Sports Medicine. Before each game or session, medical personnel should remind themselves of the basic principles of virtuous practice and the paramount importance of player autonomy.

The team doctor is often a part of the management group and has an important role to ensure that ethical principles do not get overlooked in the pursuit of victory. It is imperative that a degree of professional distance is maintained in order to achieve this. Leaders in sports medicine have advocated securing the independence of health care professionals from the club and other sporting organizations that employ them. They have also promoted the establishment of a forum between health care professionals from different organizations to facilitate discourse on ethical and professional

---

Box 1
Guidelines for the sports medical personnel

Passion for the sport—passion for the player's well-being

Dispassion in the execution of medical duties

Maintain a degree of professional distance from the management team

Informed consent is trickier in a highly charged game environment

Clear lines of reporting must be in place

Doctor first—team doctor second

Do not abdicate your responsibility to the individual player

From Devitt BM, McCarthy C. 'I am in blood Stepp'd in so far…': ethical dilemmas and the sports team doctor. Br J Sports Med 2010;44(3):177; with permission.

issues in a nonjudgmental setting.[25] Within a sporting organization, it is important to have a clearly defined medical structure to enable the medical personnel to report to a clinical colleague outside the team-management structure.[3] This clearly defined medical structure is protective not only for the player but also for the team management, the team doctor, and ultimately, the sporting organization, when ethical conflicts arise in the future.

SUMMARY

"A fit player is better than an injured star"
Sport medicine is conducted in a highly charged environment where ethical decision-making can be extremely challenging. To be an effective advocate for the players, medical personnel must remember at all times the importance of ethical medical practice, virtuousness, and professional conduct. At the end of the game, the only result that really matters is that the player's autonomy has been respected.

REFERENCES

1. Johnson R. The unique ethics of sports medicine. Clin Sports Med 2004;23(2): 175–82.
2. Bernstein J, Perlis C, Bartolozzi AR. Ethics in sports medicine. Clin Orthop Relat Res 2000;(378):50–60.
3. Devitt BM, McCarthy C. 'I am in blood Stepp'd in so far…': ethical dilemmas and the sports team doctor. Br J Sports Med 2010;44(3):175–8.
4. Lane P. The business of sport: fun, games and money. The Economist 2008.
5. Forbes list - highest paid athletes. 2015. Available at: http://www.forbes.com/ athletes/. Accessed July 8, 2015.
6. Dunn WR, George MS, Churchill L, et al. Ethics in sports medicine. Am J Sports Med 2007;35(5):840–4.
7. Brain P. Galen on the Ideal of the Physician. S Afr Med J 1977;52(23):936–8.
8. General Medical Council. Good Medical Practice - Duties of a doctor. 2015.
9. Misselbrook D. Duty, Kant, and deontology. Br J Gen Pract 2013;63(609):211.
10. Kant I, Paton HJ. The moral law: Kant's groundwork of the metaphysic of morals. New York: Barnes & Noble; 1967. p. 142.
11. Scheffler S. Consequentialism and its critics. Oxford (United Kingdom); New York: Oxford University Press; 1988. p. vi, 294.
12. Fairbank TJ. Knee joint changes after meniscectomy. J Bone Joint Surg Br 1948; 30B(4):664–70.
13. Starke C, Kopf S, Petersen W, et al. Meniscal repair. Arthroscopy 2009;25(9): 1033–44.
14. Federation International de Medecine Sportive. Principles and ethical guidelines for health care for sports medicine. Available at: http://www.fims.org/en/general/ code-of-ethics. Accessed July 8, 2015.
15. Pelligrino ED. Rationing health care: the ethics of medical gatekeeping. J Contemp Health Law Policy 1986;2:23–45.
16. Gillon R. Medical ethics: four principles plus attention to scope. BMJ 1994; 309(6948):184–8.
17. World Anti-Doping Agency. WADA Prohibited List 2015. Available at: http://list. wada-ama.org. Accessed July 8, 2015.
18. Orchard JW, Steet E, Massey A, et al. Long-term safety of using local anesthetic injections in professional rugby league. Am J Sports Med 2010;38(11):2259–66.

19. Orchard JW. Benefits and risks of using local anaesthetic for pain relief to allow early return to play in professional football. Br J Sports Med 2002;36(3):209–13.

20. World Rugby. Player welfare - Anaesthetics - Subsection 53. 2015. Available at: http://playerwelfare.worldrugby.org/?subsection=53. Accessed July 8, 2015.

21. Gardiner P. A virtue ethics approach to moral dilemmas in medicine. J Med Ethics 2003;29(5):297–302.

22. Paniagua C. Metaphysics, innateness and Plato's/Socrates' method. Int J Psychoanal 1989;70(Pt 3):549–50.

23. Beauchamp TL, Childress JF. Principles of biomedical ethics. 7th edition. New York: Oxford University Press; 2013. p. xvi, 459.

24. MacIntyre AC. After virtue: a study in moral theory. 3rd edition. Notre Dame (IN): University of Notre Dame Press; 2007. p. xix, 286.

25. Holm S, McNamee M. Ethics in sports medicine. BMJ 2009;339:b3898.

Confidentiality in Sports Medicine

Dominic Malcolm, BA, MA, PhD

KEYWORDS

- Ethics • Confidentiality • Sports medicine • Practice • Policy recommendations

KEY POINTS

- Although ethical principles identify ideal practice, ethics are always operationalized in a social context, and understanding that context is necessary for facilitating best practice.
- Sports clinicians work in a context that, if not unique, is distinct from many other areas of medical practice.
- The maintenance of confidentiality is shaped by the multiple obligations, physical environments, and practice and policy contexts of sports medicine.
- Empirical research shows that there is considerable diversity of practice in relation to maintaining patient confidentiality in sports medicine.
- A variety of policy recommendations have been made that could enable greater conformity to medical ethical best practice.

It is often claimed that the ethical challenges of sports medicine are unique.[1-4] Although claims to uniqueness may be overstated,[5] the peculiarity of sports medicine is clearly shown by the challenges of maintaining patient confidentiality. Confidentiality has been identified as one of the most important ethical issues in sports medicine,[4,6] and has been empirically shown to be among the ethical dilemmas most frequently encountered by sports doctors.[7]

Initial analyses of confidentiality in sports medicine emerged because of a belief that the specific context of sport problematized compliance with ethical practice. However, these early works were overwhelmingly personal reflections, primarily related to individuals' experiences and particular sports, and thus largely anecdotal.[8] In contrast, this article provides a more systematic and comprehensive understanding, through an overview and synthesis of existing literature. Specifically, it:

- Outlines the medical ethical principle of confidentiality and identifies cross-cultural ethicolegal variations.
- Explores 4 factors specific to the context of sport that shape the application of patient confidentiality.

Disclosure: The author has nothing to disclose.
School of Sport, Exercise and Health Sciences, Loughborough University, Epinal Way, Loughborough, Leicestershire LE11 3TU, UK
E-mail address: d.e.malcolm@lboro.ac.uk

- Reviews existing research that details practical experiences of maintaining patient confidentiality in sport.
- Summarizes the many policy recommendations that have been made for enabling and enhancing compliance with ethical practice.

THE PRINCIPLES OF CONFIDENTIALITY AND ETHICOLEGAL VARIATIONS

Historically the sovereignty of patient confidentiality has been central to medical ethics. It is the concluding item of the Hippocratic oath. The importance of confidentiality stems from the notion that doctors should work wholly and exclusively on behalf of their patients and thus it is inextricably linked to privacy, patient autonomy, and informed consent. However, it is ethical to share information with other medical providers directly involved in the patient's health care if that information is pertinent to treatment.[9] Five further mitigating circumstances that might necessitate nonconsented disclosure can be identified: incapacity of a patient; medical emergency; legal obligation to state law (but not sport-specific regulations, and hence the physician has no ethical obligation to disclose athletes' use of performance-enhancing drugs); protecting the patient's health and wellbeing; and protecting a third party from serious harm.[10]

Despite this, the literature has frequently identified the difficulties of simply transplanting medical ethical conventions into sports medicine.[2] Although some clinicians explain this by locating sports medicine as a form of occupational medicine,[11] even the Faculty of Occupational Medicine views patient confidentiality as a primary ethical issue,[12] and most ethical codes for sports medicine explicitly state that they add detail to, rather than replace, more widely recognized medical ethical principles.[13,14] The Code of Ethics published by the Fédération de Médecine du Sport explicitly states that "The physician's duty to the athlete must be his/her first concern and contractual and other responsibilities are of secondary importance."[15]

Perceptions of ethical differences have led to a correlative tendency in the literature to highlight the importance of clearly distinguishing between what has variously been termed the primary general practitioner and contracted medical official,[9] the personal and team physician,[16] and the therapeutic and assessment roles of sports medicine.[14] For instance, Bernstein and colleagues[16] argue that team physicians are obliged to work in the interests of the (sports) organization that employs them, whereas personal physicians are unequivocally devoted to individual patients (as an aside, it is debatable whether any doctor always works solely in the interests of patients uninfluenced by, for instance, budgetary constraints). However, being a team physician does not dissipate all obligations to patient confidentiality. Although team physicians are ethically obliged to prevent harm to other team members (eg, informing them of another players' infectious disease), this does not necessarily extend to a more individual issue, such as an athlete's alcohol misuse.[2] The use of the term "physician covering the team" rather than "team physician" has been proposed to clarify the obligations the role should entail.[4]

Although these terminological differences are widely discussed, their implications are variously interpreted. The views expressed by British and Australasian investigators and ethics codes are that the medical officer/team physician/assessment role is discrete in practice. In contrast, North American investigators imply that this term encompasses almost all of sports physicians' practice and that, because patients autonomously and voluntarily associate with teams, they thereby accept their rules regarding information disclosure.[4] It has been argued that, because there can be no confidentiality in sports medicine, team physicians' only alternative is to make athletes aware of their obligation to share information with other medical, coaching, and institutional personnel.[17]

This difference can partly be explained by the particular legal structure in the United States under which physicians are bound by two specific laws.[18] According to the Health Insurance Portability and Accountability Act athletes' medical records may be deemed to be part of their employment records rather than privileged health information and thus can be shared within (but not outside) the employing organization.[6] Second, the Federal Education Rights and Privacy Act (FERPA) allows disclosure of medical information with those who have an educational interest (ie, not with the media or third parties, but potentially with athletic trainers whose status is ambiguous in this respect).[2] Because ethical codes operate within legal systems that are primarily state bounded, cross-cultural variations in the maintenance of confidentiality inevitably exist. Ultimately, "the idea of a universal code … of sports medicine ethics is almost certainly a pipe dream."[5]

These cross-cultural differences illustrate a key sociological point about professions and their ethical codes. Ethical principles, although designed and claimed to be universal and immutable, operate in social contexts that are variable and dynamic. Sociologically considered medical ethics exist because of the social function they perform for the profession; namely bolstering the sense of trustworthiness and reliability that enables medicine to wield significant social power.[19] Ethical principles that hamper the influence of the medical profession are modified or discarded. Thus, aside from legal differences, it is important to consider the sport-specific contextual factors that influence the way patient confidentiality is operated in practice.

CONTEXTUAL FACTORS INFLUENCING CONFIDENTIALITY IN SPORTS MEDICINE

In identifying the following factors the aim is not to legitimize behavior that can be seen to compromise best practice, but to understand the social constraints on the operationalization of the ethical principles of patient confidentiality. Four main factors specific to the sports medicine context can be identified.

Multiple and Conflicting Obligations

Sports medicine physicians are likely to experience multiple and conflicting obligations caused by (1) sports organizations being the employers of medical personnel; (2) the competitive aspirations of players overriding health concerns; and (3) the cost of injury prevention relative to short-term and long-term morbidity.[6] This conflict has led the doctor-patient dyad to be reconceptualized in sport as the doctor-patient-team triad.[2] Conflicts of interest arise over the different priorities and values of the respective parties, and are complicated by the peculiar economic/contractual relations in sports medicine. For instance, doctors are frequently motivated by fandom[20] or ego and social status.[1] In some cases physicians pay significant amounts of money for the privilege of working with a professional sports team.[2] These factors contribute to the powerlessness of physicians within the sports context, manifest in the prominence of behaviors that serve to build trust and demonstrate usefulness.[21] Sports medicine has consequently been conceptualized as a "clients dependent practice."[22]

Physical Environment

Because sports are particularly hazardous workplaces in which injury is common, it is inevitable that some medical care is delivered in front of fellow athletes, coaches, and so forth. Such situations may be health-related emergencies, but others may only be emergencies in the context of sports performance. This environment may therefore expose clinicians to well-meaning questions from concerned teammates[23] and stimulate management demands for prognoses. The openness of sports medicine treatment is compounded by the design of treatment facilities in sport, which conventionally have little regard for athlete-patients' privacy.[7,24]

Moreover, sports medicine may be practiced on the playing field in front of thousands of spectators. This situation fuels a widespread misconception that information about athletes' injuries is public knowledge. Orchard[25] seemingly views the nonexistence of privacy as an inconsequential "side effect of the enormous pay packet afforded to a professional football player" and is sanguine about the circumvention of patient confidentiality issues, arguing that as "part of the entertainment ... in this sense no one 'owns' the information."[25] Although this position is directly counter to (sports) medical ethical codes, it is clear that the accessibility of information about athletes' medical conditions creates a distinct environmental context that constrains clinicians' maintenance of patient confidentiality.

An additional but increasingly important feature of the physical environment of sports medicine is the media. Although much potentially sensitive medical information is benignly disseminated, journalists are also malignantly proactive in this process. In 1980, Peter Sperryn[8] complained about the "constant pryings of the media" and information leaks from "hospital switchboards,"[8] but the expansion of media outlets (eg, the Internet) has heightened this issue. Consequently medical information appears throughout the media and although there may be multiple sources for that information, the pressures on clinical staff to release confidential patient data are considerable.[26] In an age in which professional reputations and commercial value are fostered via social media, the incentives to act unethically are increased.[27]

Practice Context

Sports medicine is fundamentally a multidisciplinary practice. For instance, Ryan[28] has argued that sports medicine practitioners may include "physicians, coaches, trainers, exercise physiologists, psychologists, sociologists, physical educators and others whose special interests are less well-defined."[28] Clinicians therefore tend to work in multidisciplinary sport science teams (MSSTs) alongside colleagues whose degree of training, familiarity, and concordance with medical ethical principles varies. "With so many differences between disciplines, how is the athlete to distinguish who says what to whom?"[29]

The adversarial nature of sports medicine practice further complicates confidentiality issues. Elite sport entails continuous experimentation on the human body assessed through physical competition. Athletes are subject to on-going performance testing, from GPS (global positioning system) tracking to the monitoring and assessment of supplement use. Medical staff are varyingly engaged in these performance-based activities; the American College of Sports Medicine's Team Physician Consensus Statement argues that it is essential that team physicians embrace performance issues.[18] Health care personnel may even be included in performance-based financial reward systems.[22] Thus the medical and nonmedical spheres in the practice environment of sport are frequently blurred. Further complicating confidentiality issues therefore is the frequency with which individuals perform roles that span both health care and performance.

The complexities of sports medicine's practice context are evident in the system of transferring athletes between clubs, or from colleges to professional teams. This system creates gray areas regarding confidentiality. Given the speed with which many transfers occur, it is often impossible to get signed and informed consent from a player to release confidential medical information. Player movement raises the question of what information is owned by the sports organization (eg, results of particular interventions) and what belongs to the player? Moreover, what is the duty of the club/college to disclose the medical condition of the asset they are releasing?[6] In addition, consider the aborted transfer of Ruud van Nistelrooy in 2000 because of concerns revealed during the medical conducted by the purchasing club. The abandoned transfer became a global news story, but who released that information?

Policy Context

Sports physicians work within the constraints of a variety of sports-specific policies that require the routine disclosure of otherwise privileged information. Although it can be assumed that athletes largely consent to these disclosures, their choices are highly constrained by their desire to participate in sport. Policies relating to the screening and policing of sports participants are particularly problematic.

Testing for performance-enhancing drugs has been widely criticized for infringing the basic human right to privacy on which the ethical principle of confidentiality is based. Although such testing is frequently justified on the grounds that it prevents harm to individuals, safeguards equality, and is in the economic interests of sport, the most ethically challenging issues relate to:

- The whereabouts system, which requires athletes to disclose their movements to enable no-notice, out-of-competition testing.
- Testing for recreational drugs, such as marijuana, that do not have performance-enhancing potential, but the use of which may be deemed to bring the sport into disrepute.
- The therapeutic use exemption system, in which athletes must declare their use of medications that may otherwise lead to positive tests (and thus potentially disclose medical conditions).[30]

The conflict between these drug-related policies and patient confidentiality is most clearly evident in the 2009 World Anti-Doping Code. This code stipulates that clinicians are themselves guilty of a doping offense if they do not report athletes' illegal drug use, even when that action is in contravention of their ethical duty to preserve patient confidentiality.[31]

The procedures required to maintain sex segregation in sport further entail the public disclosure of medical evaluations. The case of Caster Semenya showed that, based on little more than suspicion borne of visual impression, athletes could be subject to extensive medical and media scrutiny. Although the detail of what the investigations found is not known, the outcome (that she qualifies to participate as a woman) is public knowledge. Similar issues relate to the criteria governing the participation of transsexuals in sport as outlined by the International Olympic Committee's Stockholm Consensus. Sex segregation in sport necessarily entails the public dissemination of medical information that would otherwise be considered privileged and subject to patient confidentiality.[32]

Concerns have been expressed that cardiac screening, even when voluntary, may represent a coercive offer and so contravene the notion of informed consent.[33] However, policies that entail both mandatory testing and the enforced cessation of competitive sport (for athletes who test positive) are also problematic from a confidentiality point of view. Although it may be argued that such policies are designed to protect individuals from harm, the resistance of some athletes who have been forced to withdraw from sport following such tests raises questions about the ethicality of this practice.

In conclusion, sports participation regulations frequently entail the public dissemination of privileged medical information (other examples include the prefight and postfight assessment of boxers, and the classification of athletes with disabilities). This policy environment is becoming more complex as diagnostic technology improves. For instance, concerns have been raised in relation to the potential of genetic testing, which will require clarification regarding with whom data can be shared, and inevitably affects the privacy of relatives.[34] In a context in which such information is routinely shared, people are likely to become desensitized to patients' right to confidentiality.

OPERATIONALIZING PATIENT CONFIDENTIALITY IN SPORT

Several studies have examined how the medical profession, professions allied to medicine, and other people who work in MSSTs operationalize confidentiality in sport. Three studies have focused on doctors and physiotherapists in elite/professional sport, and a further five have concentrated on a wider range of health care professions, primarily in North American college sport. Comparison of health care in professional and college sport shows different emphases on the culture of risk and the culture of precaution, which shape return-to-play decisions (often a key site for confidentiality conflicts).[35] It has also been argued that athletes in individual sports are less open to the sharing of medical information than those in team sports.[23] These and other variations affect how clinicians working in sport deal with patient confidentiality in their everyday practice.

Anderson and colleagues[7,36] explored the ethical issues concerning New Zealand sports doctors. A half of respondents stated that they were contractually bound to disclose information to coaching staff and a third stated that they had disclosed information that athletes wished to remain confidential (examples related to infectious disease, the use of performance-enhancing and pain relieving medication, and pregnancy). They expressed concerns that (1) many coaches are unaware of the ethical constraints on clinicians to uphold patient confidentiality; (2) sports organizations frequently do not have clear lines of communication; and thus (3) controlling the flow of medical information is difficult. Athletes were also often contractually bound to waive the right to confidentiality.[37]

The research revealed a high level of inconsistency among sports physicians. Most doctors stated that they would defy their contractual obligations and withhold information from coaches because of the perceived higher ethical duty and practical importance of establishing patients' trust. Alternatively, to avoid conflict they might provide coaches with limited or partial information. Interviewees found the preservation of confidentiality in relation to performance-related information especially challenging.[38]

In addition, this research also highlighted the media pressures related to confidentiality. Sports physicians described being continually pestered by journalists who had no regard for patient confidentiality. Experiences of media coercion included threats to fabricate stories if factual information was not provided.[7] Respondents sought to alleviate these pressures by, for example, drip-feeding information or repeating what was already known. However, they also revealed an awareness of the interdependence between injury reports; media exposure for a commercial franchise; the value of sponsorship rights; and, ultimately, clinicians' own economic interests.[36]

Waddington and Roderick[12] identified a similar lack of behavioral uniformity in research focused on clinicians working in professional football in the United Kingdom. Doctors and physiotherapists reported practices that ranged from strictly respecting patient privacy to an almost total disregard based on the view that it was essential and beneficial for managers to have full information access. Again, different opinions were expressed about the differences when dealing with performance and non–performance-related information (eg, player injuries as opposed to social drug use). Physiotherapists, many of whom had only base-level qualifications and, consequently, no experience of practicing in other health care settings, were perceived by doctors to be particularly culpable of breaking patient confidentiality. The investigators concluded that medical confidentiality was poorly maintained in professional football because medical staff too often thought that a coach's status gave them the right to access all information.

Uniquely, this research also incorporated athletes' views on confidentiality. Significantly, footballers routinely sought to minimize disclosure of information to medical staff because of the expectation that it would be divulged to management. Confidentiality breaches therefore had a negative impact on the quality of athletes' medical care.

Third, Malcolm and Scott's[24] research conducted with members of the British Olympic Association's Medical Committee and Physiotherapy Forum found much more consistent recognition of the privileged nature of patient information. These interviewees again reported that athletes' contracts frequently required them to waive medical confidentiality but noted that, when athletes resisted these obligations, clinicians were required to develop interpersonal strategies to minimize conflicts of interest. Strategies included:

- Persuading athletes that disclosure was in their own interests (eg, avoiding an unexplained decline in performance).
- Suggesting that upholding patient confidentiality would lead clinicians to be bypassed by coaches, leaving the athlete more exposed/isolated.
- Highlighting how the athletes' actions could harm others in the sports organization.
- Co-opting clinical colleagues to exert pressure on the athlete.
- Psychological tricks to challenge athletes' rationales for nondisclosure.

In sum, and epitomizing the variability of practice, research with elite sport clinicians shows both strong paternalism and allegations of malpractice. Waddington and Roderick[12] reported how a physiotherapist falsified information in order to protect a footballer with an alcohol problem,[12] whereas Anderson[37] relayed clinicians' stories of creating fictitious physical injuries to obscure athletes' mental health issues. These reports mirror findings regarding clinicians' avoidance of concussion diagnoses in order to obviate conflict with athletes and coaches.[39] In contrast, in a serious case of alleged malpractice, a footballer recalled a doctor threatening to release confidential medical information (which turned out to be false) in order to dissuade the player from seeking a lucrative transfer.[12]

Five further studies have focused on the attitudes and behaviors of practitioners incorporated in MSSTs.

Sports Psychologists

Reid and colleagues'[40] account of psychologists' experiences of working to establish an effective MSST focuses on the everyday challenges of confidentiality. They identify differing communication protocols (including regarding confidentiality), driven by conflicts between the needs of individual athletes and the wider group, as a potential barrier to success. Their proposed solution rested on persuading athletes to permit full disclosure of personal data, effectively ignoring the rights of patients to confidentiality.

Complementing this study is Andersen's[41] view that reports of serious confidentiality breaches among sports psychologists "are all too common."[41] He notes that some disclosure may be linked to the constraints of certain national sports systems or legal requirements, or may be a consequence of the conflicts of interest stemming from working with teams. However, significant harm is done to the profession by unlicensed, unchartered, or unregistered "sports psychologists" who "routinely violate" the principles of confidentiality, including disclosing the names of celebrity clients to enhance their social and commercial status.

Athletic Trainers

Research focusing on this group reveals confidentiality issues to be perceived as infrequent,[42] or as recurrent, important, but largely manageable.[23] Many athletic trainers reported that student-athletes were required to sign consent waivers but that any subsequent confidentiality conflicts that occurred could be dealt with by (1) challenging individuals to allow them to disclose; (2) being vague or partial in information disclosure; (3) contacting colleagues/mentors for advice; and (4) seeking support elsewhere in the university. Student athletic therapists who, as peers, were more likely to be friends with the athletes they treated experienced particularly blurred practice boundaries. However, the controllable nature of these issues was attributed to the lesser economic pressures of the sport, which in turn lessened pressures from and conflicts with the media. In addition, athletic trainers' contractual arrangements with universities rather than individual teams, and the legal regulations related to FERPA, may also be significant.

Fitness Professionals

An Australian study revealed that this group received limited training in professional ethics, which resulted, in part, in a variety of behaviors regarding confidentiality.[43] Specifically, large numbers (mistakenly) thought that sharing client data with colleagues and other gym members, and reporting suspicions of illegal substance use to criminal authorities, were ethically acceptable practices.

Combined, empirical studies show that the reality of operationalizing confidentiality in sport involves a wide variety of practice between as well as within professions.

RECOMMENDATIONS

In light of the practical experiences of patient confidentiality in sports medicine, five categories of policy recommendations have been made.

Roles

Various investigators recommend the clear separation of different sports medicine roles.[3,5,38] For those whose work is akin to occupational medicine (eg, working as a team physician or in an assessment role) there is a clearer (but not unequivocal) case to be subject to full disclosure. In contrast, those acting as general practitioners in therapeutic roles should maintain the highest ethical levels in relation to patient confidentiality. Although a shortage of appropriately qualified and motivated personnel is acknowledged, ideally no individual should occupy multiple roles. To this end, some investigators recommend not only that players should have a primary physician outside of sport but that sports organizations should encourage and enable athletes in this regard.[4,20] The broader legal framework affects the appropriateness and feasibility of role separation.

Clarity

Building on the principle of informed consent, role separation requires that clinicians and athletes fully understand the health care system in which they operate.[38] For some investigators, this requires transparent reporting and information management systems.[5] Other investigators have advocated the use of an athlete's charter to identify the MSST personnel who are bound by disclosure regulations.[4,29] A dialogue to establish what is deemed to constitute serious harm to third parties within sports teams is required because research identifies various interpretations of this notion.[24] Clarifying the appropriate balance of individual and group interests may alleviate pressures to disclose confidential information. Robust ethical codes are essential to adding clarity.[37]

Contracts

Although written agreements contribute to clarity of expectation, most researchers have warned against their use. For instance, it has been argued that the contractual obligations of sports physicians should be limited to reduce the conflict between occupational expectations and medical ethical principles.[37] Similarly, athletes' consent to disclose must be specific rather than general, the exception not the norm, and must be free of any element of coercion.[5,24] Research shows that such contracts are redundant because both doctors and athletes consistently disregard their terms with seemingly limited sanction.

Education

In recognition of the variability in practice it is the duty of clinicians to ensure that they keep themselves updated on current ethical standards.[4] Calls have been made for sports organizations to develop and disseminate models of good practice,[12] and enhance confidentiality-based continuous professional development.[24] Wider educational provision for sports psychologists[41] and coaching/training staff[4] has also been advocated, which should be extended to all members of MSSTs.

Facilities

The provision of medical facilities that safeguard and/or maximize patient privacy has been recommended.[24]

SUMMARY

Ethics refers to idealized codes of behavior and consequently sports medicine ethics cannot be seen as unique or subject to lesser standards. However, it is true that the social context in which sports medicine ethics are operationalized has distinct characteristics and manifestly structures the behavior of those charged with the duty to act ethically. Studies of the practice of maintaining patient confidentiality in sports medicine show, for example, that the distinct physical environment, practice, and policy context of sports medicine, and the conflicts of interest that stem from multiple obligations, shape how patient confidentiality is maintained. Breaches in confidentiality are common and there is considerable variation within and between professional groups regarding the maintenance of patient confidentiality. However, there are a variety of actions that could be taken to bolster ethical practice in sport in relation to patient confidentiality and this implementation is vital to uphold the status and influence of sports medicine and the various related professions that populate MSSTs.

REFERENCES

1. Bernstein J, Perlis C, Bartolozzi AR. Ethics in sports medicine. Clin Orthop Relat Res 2000;(378):50–60.

2. Dunn SR, George MS, Churchill L, et al. Ethics in sports medicine. Am J Sports Med 2007;35:840–4.
3. Devitt BM, McCarthy C. "I am in blood Stepp'd in so far...": ethical dilemmas and the sports team doctor. Br J Sports Med 2010;44:175–8.
4. Testoni D, Hornik C, Smith PB, et al. Sports medicine and ethics. The Am J Bioeth 2013;13(10):4–12.
5. Holm S, McNamee M, Pigozzi F. Ethical practice and sports physician protection: a proposal. Br J Sports Med 2011;45:1170–3.
6. Stovitz SD, Satin DJ. Professionalism and the ethics of the sideline physician. Curr Sports Med Rep 2006;5:120–4.
7. Anderson L, Gerrard DF. Ethical issues concerning New Zealand sports doctors. J Med Ethics 2005;31:88–92.
8. Sperryn P. Ethics in sports medicine – the sports physician. Br J Sports Med 1980;14(2/3):84–9.
9. Faculty of Sport and Exercise Medicine. Professional code. Edinburgh (United Kingdom): Faculty of Sport and Exercise Medicine; 2009.
10. Exercise and Sports Science Australia. Code of professional conduct and ethical practice. Queensland (Australia): Exercise and Sports Science Australia; 2014.
11. Crane J. Association football: the team doctor. In: Payne SDW, editor. Medicine, sport and the law. Oxford (United Kingdom): Blackwell Scientific Publications; 1990. p. 331–7.
12. Wadddington I, Roderick M. Management of medical confidentiality in English professional football clubs: some ethical problems and issues. Br J Sports Med 2002;36:118–23.
13. British Olympic Association. The British Olympic Association's position statement on athlete confidentiality. Br J Sports Med 2000;34:71–2.
14. Australasian College of Sports Physicians' code of ethics and professional behaviour. New Zealand J Sports Med 2013;40(1):43.
15. FIMS. Code of ethics. Available at: http://www.fims.org/files/8214/1933/5848/FIMSCodeOfEthics.pdf. Accessed July 1, 2015.
16. Bernstein J, Perlis C, Bartolozzi AR. Normative ethics in sports medicine. Clin Orthop Relat Res 2004;420:309–18.
17. Johnson R. The unique ethics of sports medicine. Clin Sports Med 2004;23(2):175–82.
18. Herring SA, Kibler WB, Putukian M. Team physician consensus statement: 2013 update. Med Sci Sports Exerc 2013;45(8):1618–22.
19. MacDonald KM. The sociology of the professions. London: Sage; 1995.
20. Wadddington I, Roderick M, Parker G. Managing injuries in professional football: a study of the roles of the club doctor and physiotherapist. Leicester (United Kingdom): Centre for Research into Sport and Society; 1999.
21. Malcolm D, Scott A. "Involved in every step": how working practices shape the influence of physiotherapists in elite sport. Qualitative Research in Sport, Exercise and Health 2015;7(4–5):539–57.
22. Malcolm D. Unprofessional practice? The power and status of sports physicians. Sociol Sport J 2006;23(4):376–95.
23. Riendeau C, Parent-Houle V, Legel-Gariel ME, et al. An investigation of how university sports team athletic therapists and physical therapists experience ethical issues. J Orthop Sports Phys Ther 2015;45(3):198–206.
24. Malcolm D, Scott A. Practical responses to confidentiality dilemmas in elite sport medicine. Br J Sports Med 2013;48(19):1410–3.
25. Orchard J. Who owns the information? Br J Sports Med 2002;36:16–8.

26. Ribbans B, Ribbans H, Nightingale C, et al. Sports medicine, confidentiality and the press. Br J Sports Med 2013;47:40–3.
27. Sports Physiotherapy New Zealand. Sports physiotherapy code of conduct, 2013. Available at: http://sportsphysiotherapy.org.nz/sportsphysiotherapy.org.nz/documents/Sports-Physiotherapy-Code-of-Conduct.pdf. Accessed July 1, 2015.
28. Ryan AJ. Sports medicine in the world today. In: Ryan AJ, Allman FL, editors. Sports medicine. 2nd edition. San Diego (CA): Academic Press; 1989. p. 13.
29. Collins D, Moore P, Mitchell D, et al. Role conflict and confidentiality in multidisciplinary athlete support programmes. Br J Sports Med 1999;33:208–11.
30. Schneider AJ. Privacy, confidentiality and human rights in sport. Sport Soc 2004; 7(3):438–56.
31. McNamee M, Phillips N. Confidentiality, disclosure and doping in sports medicine. Br J Sports Med 2011;45:174–7.
32. Caplan AL. Fairer sex: The ethics of determining gender for athletic ability. J Genet Counsel 2010;19:549–50.
33. Anderson L, Exeter D, Bowyer L. Sudden cardiac death: mandatory exclusion of athletes at risk is a step too far. Br J Sports Med 2012;46:331–4.
34. McNamee MJ, Müller A, van Hilvoorde I, et al. Genetic testing and sports medicine ethics. Sports Med 2009;39(5):339–44.
35. Safai P. Healing the body in the "culture of risk": Examining the negotiations of treatment between sport medicine clinicians and injured athletes in Canadian intercollegiate sport. Sociol Sport J 2003;20:127–46.
36. Anderson L, Jackson S. Competing loyalties in sports medicine: Threats to medical professionalism in elite commercial sport. Int Rev Soc Sport 2012;48(2):238–56.
37. Anderson L. Writing a new code of ethics for sports physicians: principles and challenges. Br J Sports Med 2009;43:1079–82.
38. Anderson L. Contractual obligations and the sharing of confidential health information in sport. J Med Ethics 2008;34:e6.
39. Malcolm D. Medical uncertainty and clinician-athlete relations: the management of concussion injuries in rugby union. Sociol Sport J 2009;26(2):191–210.
40. Reid C, Stewart E, Thorne G. Multidisciplinary sport science teams in elite sport. The Sport Psychol 2004;18:204–17.
41. Andersen M. "Yeah I work with Beckham": Issues of confidentiality, privacy and privilege in sport psychology service delivery. Sp Ex Psyc Rev 2005;1(2):5–13.
42. Swisher LL, Nyland J, Klossner D, et al. Ethical issues in athletic training: a foundational descriptive investigation. Athletic Ther Today 2006;14(2):3–9.
43. Dawson A, Andersen MB, Hemphill D. The ethical beliefs and behaviours of Victorian fitness professionals. J Sci Med Sport 2001;4(3):266–82.

Conflicts of Interest in Sports Medicine

Andrew M. Tucker, MD

KEYWORDS

- Sports medicine • Confidentiality • Conflicts of interest

KEY POINTS

- Confidentiality, a fundamental to the practice of medicine, is altered by the team physician's dual responsibilities to the player-patient and the team.
- Documents constructed by the team generally specify the parameters by which health information may be handled.
- Oftentimes, these ground rules are not truly understood by the player or the clinician.
- Even in the best of circumstances, situations will arise that will challenge the clinician's judgment as to handling of confidential health information.
- The team doctor should make a strong effort to understand the rules of handling personal health information, and seek to discuss these issues with both the player-patients and team administration in hopes of preempting or minimizing conflicts.
- Clinical decision making in sports medicine may manifest conflicts of competing interests – short term pursuits of competition and success versus long term health.
- Team physicians must assist the player-patient in determining their priorities, and be aware of other influences that may negatively affect the pursuit of the primary interest(s).

Although society generally expects physicians to act only in their patient's best interests, sports medicine, especially at the highest competitive levels, can produce circumstances that threaten the exclusive commitment to the patient.[1] As has been pointed out, challenges in the areas of conflict of interest (COI), confidentiality, consent, and disclosure are not exclusive to the arena of sports medicine, but still may be considered as unique in their presentation and more consistently prevalent in the sports physician's practice.[2] The goals of this article were to review the evolution of professional team physician relationships, the definition and concepts of COI, expand on the issues of potential COI that confront sports medicine physicians, particularly at the professional and major college level of competition, and offer observations of this topic from personal experiences in caring for a professional sports team.

Although this topic always has long generated interest, the controversies in the past several years surrounding concussion diagnosis, management, and possible long-term complications, has magnified the scrutiny of team physician clinical decision

Medstar Union Memorial Sports Medicine, 1407 York Road, Suite 100A, Lutherville, MD 21093, USA
E-mail address: Andrew.Tucker@medstar.net

Clin Sports Med 35 (2016) 217–226
http://dx.doi.org/10.1016/j.csm.2015.10.010
0278-5919/16/$ – see front matter © 2016 Elsevier Inc. All rights reserved.
sportsmed.theclinics.com

making in the context of influences on both patient and provider, and the threat of conflicts on those decisions.

HISTORY

Many years ago, team physician positions, especially at the professional level, were often the product of convenience and personal relationships. Before medical specialization and fellowship training, professional team doctors were often friends or acquaintances of the team owner. The physician was not necessarily skilled in the care of athletic injuries or exercise science. Needless to say, this type of medical care arrangement likely presented overt conflicts of interest, with medical decisions easily scrutinized and potentially influenced by the physician's friend/owner.

During the 1980s and 1990s, the field of sports medicine evolved into a distinct specialty, an entity populated by fellowship-trained orthopedic surgeons and primary care physicians. Combined with the burgeoning "big business" of professional and major college sports, the need for highly trained and experienced clinicians who were more capable of evaluation and treatment of high-level athletes became necessary. Team physicians were selected for specific skills and experience and less likely to be friends of the owner or a university athletic director, and thus less likely to be easily influenced by the boss. Although this arrangement is clearly a better model for the delivery of care to a sports team and its participants, it is not devoid of COI issues.

One physician explained it this way: "...in the 1990s professional and college sports teams became big business, with escalating salaries and increased emphasis on winning, sometimes at all costs. Corporations began acquiring teams, and players sought counsel from agents, lawyers, and other advisors who wanted a position in the decision tree. The role of the team physician became decidedly different."[3]

It is safe to say the environment in which sports medicine physicians make clinical decisions has become more complex, and likewise, so are the decisions that must be made regarding their player-patient. The list of potential distractions and influences include the pervasive media presence in our society, the high dollar value of contracts (and college tuitions for scholastic athletes), the existence of medical sponsorships, the heightened visibility and prestige being attached to team physician roles, and so on.

In a more perfect world, guidance for the physician would be available to assist in navigating these many challenges. There are relatively few substantive guidelines for team doctors to help deal with the potential conflicts between pressure to win and the standards of medical ethics.[4] Codes of conduct have been promulgated by various organizations over the years (American College of Sports Medicine [ACSM], Australasian College of Sports Medicine [ACSP], Federation Internationale de Medicine Sportive [FIMS], Faculty of Sport and Exercise Medicine [FASEM]),[5] but the value to a clinician is seen as limited.[2] Years ago, the ACSM offered this general advice to team doctors: "when confronted by pressures from coaches and athletes, the team physician has the obligation to put those pressures aside when providing treatment."[4]

CONFLICT OF INTEREST CONCEPTS

COIs are prevalent in our medical system, starting with the nature of reimbursement, where clinicians may be financially rewarded for doing more (or less, depending on the system). The pharmaceutical and medical equipment industries seek to influence the practice patterns of physicians. Medical research itself can be influenced by the source of support or funding.

Before reviewing COIs in sports medicine, it is appropriate to establish a framework of understanding of its concepts. One definition of COI is defined as a set of circumstances that creates a risk that professional judgment or actions regarding a primary interest will be unduly influenced by a secondary interest. Thus, there are 3 main elements required for a COI to exist: a primary interest, a secondary interest, and the conflict.[6]

It has been pointed out that whatever the primary interests may be, the goal of regulating COI is to try to ensure that the secondary interests do not subvert or undermine a physician's decision and actions regarding the primary interest. It also should be pointed out that primary interests sometimes conflict with each other, for example, the long-term health of an individual, and that individual's desire to attain an athletic scholarship that will provide the means for a college education.[6]

Secondary interests are not necessarily "bad," and are frequently legitimate and even desirable goals. They are problematic only when they exert greater weight than the primary interest in decision making. Undue influence can be thought of as when the secondary interest distorts the pursuit of the primary interest.[6]

Conflict is the third necessary element. It exists not when the primary interest is unnecessarily compromised, but rather is a set of circumstances or relationships that create or increase the risk that the primary interest will be neglected as a result of the influence or pursuit of the secondary interest.

It should be emphasized that COIs are often not easily identified, nor directly quantifiable. Financial conflicts of interest may be a common example that can be, on the surface, more readily identified and possibly quantifiable. However, such an acknowledgment by a physician does not allow for a simple judgment of the extent or magnitude of influence, or whether the circumstances result in any undue influence at all.

Other conflicts exist that can be confused with COI. For example, conflict of obligations can be defined as duties that require different actions but only one of the different actions can be taken in a given circumstance.[6] One example of conflict of obligation in general medicine is the physician's dilemma of whether to maintain confidentiality for a patient who has a contagious disease. One legitimate claim is the importance of maintaining the patient's confidentiality: divulging this information can have significant untoward consequences to the patient. The other interest to be considered is that of public health and the benefit to others by sharing this information with the appropriate parties. Both claims are legitimate primary interests, and can be thought of as essentially a conflict of primary interests.

AREAS OF LIKELY CONFLICTS

In this section, we look at 2 issues in the context of sports medicine: confidentiality and clinical decision making. Both have been identified as areas of fertile ground for potential conflict, where primary and secondary interests may be confused, and become subject to a number of influences.

Confidentiality

Confidentiality is a bedrock fundamental of medical relationship between patient and physician. Patients freely disclose information to physicians because they trust that information will be kept in confidence.[1] The freedom with which information is shared allows a treating physician to most effectively diagnose and treat.

The Health Insurance Portability and Accountability Act (HIPAA) of 1996 established standards for the medical provider's treatment of a patient's protected health information yet may not apply in employer-employee relationships.[7] In professional sports, collective bargaining agreements are likely to govern who, and to whom, a player-patient's health information may be shared.

Team physicians have obligations to the team or entity they are working for, or are representing, and as such, have contractual obligations to share certain information about a player's health with the team management.[8] Information about injuries and medical conditions can and will affect a team's perception of a player and ultimately affect the player's employability. The information is critical to a team's personnel department that is charged with incorporating information on health with the scouting and coaching assessment of skill and talent. Ideally, these responsibilities of the physician to the team or school are clearly defined by agreements to be read, understood, and signed by the player-patient. These forms delineate the ground rules for how health information is treated, specifically the content and the potential recipients of such information.

The athlete should have some understanding of the dual responsibilities that the physician has to the athlete and the professional club or university. However, the number of forms signed by an entering collegiate athlete or a newly employed professional athlete can be difficult to assimilate and may not be truly understood by the athlete. The pressures to get through the paperwork and all the other requisite obligations of athlete and medical staff do not lend themselves to a thoughtful reading and comprehension on the part of the athlete. Unfortunately, the same may be true of many clinicians: their understanding of what they can or cannot do with the athlete's medical information may be equally as hazy. However, the clinician bears the responsibility to understand what information can be shared, either with other members of the medical staff as well as nonmedical personnel with the team.

Even in "ideal" circumstances in which both clinician and athlete are reasonably well informed of the rules for sharing of medical information, there will be gray areas that will not be easily reconciled. Although professional teams or colleges may have the right to be told of injuries or conditions that will directly affect ability to practice and play (eg, musculoskeletal injury, concussion), medical conditions may exist that present a more complicated picture. When should a psychiatric condition or substance abuse problem that is known by the clinician and medical staff be shared with the team? A survey of sports medicine physicians confirmed that confidentiality of this sort was an area of likely conflict. When asked about sensitive health information (recreational drug use, blood-borne infections, use of pain-relieving medication and performance-enhancing agents), half of the respondents reported disclosing such information to team management, and half had not.[8]

It is clear that the amount and type of medical information of a player-patient that is shared with team management and coaches is likely to vary from setting to setting, and may vary even with a single physician. It is equally clear that this inconsistency, and an awareness of this fact on the part of the player-patient, does not lend itself to an environment of trust on which to build a physician and patient relationship.

Returning to our basic concepts of COI, these issues of confidentiality seem to represent the previously mentioned conflict of obligations, as much as COI. One obligation or duty is to the team, the other is to the patient, and both are legitimate. The team physician must understand and be continually sensitive to these parallel responsibilities. It is this author's sense that in cases of conflict of obligation, most clinicians seek to err on the side of the player, so as to protect the physician-patient relationship to the greatest extent possible. Doing so may put at risk the team physician's relationship with the team. Failure to protect the physician-patient relationship risks the trust and confidence of the team members in the physician.

The player-patient has a corresponding duty to disclose medical information to the team physicians. This duty is typically spelled out in the legal forms that are executed by both parties at the time of physical examination, and creates the framework for the type and amount of information to be shared with the team physicians and the club. Given the magnitude of what is frequently at stake for these individuals, they often are incentivized to withhold information from clinicians, and thus the team, so as to maximize their employability. This fact can create a tension between player and the physician at the outset of the relationship, and can contribute to undermining the trust that is critical to optimal patient care.

CLINICAL DECISION MAKING

Perhaps the most frequently visited area of conflict in sports medicine is clinical decision making, where it may not always be clear how to interpret or prioritize the "best interests of the patient."[2] Medical decisions confronting the physician and the athlete have potential implications for the short term (return to play) and the long term (risk of medical or orthopedic problems in the future), and the two may be at odds. For those who view medicine's purpose to maximize long-term health, the sports medicine environment will be uncomfortable, as it is populated by patients who have devoted their lives to pursuit of performing and winning now, or at worst, in the very near term.

For a musculoskeletal injury, a treatment or management plan that allows a more rapid return to play is often in the best interests of the team, whose success may depend on a player being on the field or court. This same approach may be in the best short-term interest of a player who is competing for a job on the team, or who is trying to secure the next longer-term contract that may mean financial security for an extended period of time. Players who spend significant time on the injury list become less attractive to their team employers. A typical example of an orthopedic injury that poses short-term versus long-term health implications is the repairable meniscus tear. The partial meniscectomy offers the patient the most expeditious return to play, likely at a cost of more rapid development of degenerative knee changes. The meniscus repair offers the athlete the better odds of preserving articular cartilage health for the long term, yet the postoperative recovery will certainly be much longer, and there remains the risk of re-tear once the player returns. The counseling approach to the patient by the physician and medical staff likely can be very influential in the athlete's decision. Other influences on the player include family and friends, agent, other players, coaches, or management.

An area of great interest in recent years is the diagnosis and management of concussion. Several case reports and small retrospective cohorts of deceased former professional athletes, many from football but including other sports and contact/collision activities, have been published that link a history of repeated concussion or repetitive head trauma (subconcussive blows) to a specific neuropathological condition that has been labeled chronic traumatic encephalopathy.[9] Although a review of this entity is not appropriate here, the controversies surrounding the evaluation and management of concussion, as well as criticism of allegedly biased research into this injury, has provided fertile ground for the examination of the conflicts that can confront player, coach, management, and medical staff.[10] For example, a player who sustains a seemingly minor concussion in an important game is adamant that he is "fine" and able to return to the contest. The primary interest of long-term player health can easily be subverted by the competing interests of doing what may be most beneficial for the team.

Likewise, a player who has sustained a number of concussions over his or her career desires to return to play. The physician is appropriately concerned about vulnerability to recurrent injury and a risk of cumulative damage that may not manifest for many years. Secondary interests of both the physician and team lurk as risks to proper pursuit of the primary interest. This all too common scenario is complicated by the absence of reliable testing that can help to properly quantitate the actual risk. How does the clinician adequately counsel and inform when there is so much unknown?

Using the previously discussed definition of COI, we can construct some virtual tables of typical primary and secondary interests, and the type and sources of potential conflict. As noted previously, the young athlete with a repairable meniscus tear sustained early in the season presents the physician with the often cited primary interest (long-term knee health), and a typical secondary interest (more expeditious return to play). The potential conflicts are plentiful: coach and/or administration in desperate need of the player's return, the athlete's soldier mentality of wanting to return to competition with his teammates as fast as possible, and a physician's desire to please everybody involved, including a fan base whose dreams of a championship season are possibly resting on the return of a certain athlete. We note the secondary interest here, a rapid return to play, is not a "bad" pursuit at all. There can be many tangible and intangible benefits of such a secondary interest. What the scenario delivers is a set of circumstances in which the secondary interests can overwhelm or distort the pursuit of the primary interest.

Note that the physician's role, as defined by our standard societal expectations, is to protect the patient's long-term health.[11] Many would consider this standard as fundamental to the practice of medicine and the lens that through which most or all medical decisions should be evaluated. This construct is relatively straightforward, and also seems to assume that the physician takes on the more traditional, paternalistic role in that he or she would be the primary arbiter of what constitutes a decision in the best interest of long-term health.

However, medicine has evolved to the place where we are today, in which the primary role of physician is now thought to be as the experienced and informed source of information for various treatment options, with the patient taking on an active role in the decision-making process.[12] The patient is presented with the pros and cons of various treatment options and makes a decision deemed best for himself or herself. The patient is more autonomous in this model, and it assumes the basic premises that the patient is competent and capable to make an informed decision.

Although we can assume a young athlete is competent and capable of decision making, some point out that frequently in sports medicine, the environment in which a player-patient makes medical decisions, given all the potential attendant pressures, is not at all conducive to a truly rational consideration of options and an informed decision. Even with complete discussion of treatment options, the athlete, in the crucible of competition and its associated influences, will not properly engage in the process. In this setting, the physician should rightfully take the active and paternalistic role in the decision-making process.[12]

If we are to look at a number of sports medicine treatment scenarios, including the case of a repairable meniscus in season, we can easily see that our virtual table of primary and secondary interests can be fluid and changeable, depending on any number of variables that are almost too numerous to mention. The player-patient becomes a primary decision maker as to what constitutes a primary and secondary interest, and these can change for the same patient. For example, a young professional athlete with a projected long and productive career ahead of him or her is perhaps more likely select career longevity and long-term competitive health as the primary interest, with rapid return to play as their secondary interest. The potential conflict, and sources of conflict, will remain, and may include coaches, fellow players, family members, agents, team administration, and an expectant fan base.

An athlete nearing the end of his or her career is likely to have an entirely different perspective: a short time period left to complete his or her playing career, one last opportunity to win a trophy, or the "ring." For this individual, the primary interest is now short-term health and rapid return to function. Long-term health becomes not unimportant, but a secondary goal. Thus, decisions about pregame use of analgesics, such as ketorolac, or periodic injections of corticosteroids can be viewed in a different light depending on such individual circumstances. If the physician determines it is appropriate to defer decisions of primary and secondary interest to the player-patient, it is incumbent on the physician to not relinquish the critical role of assisting the player-patient in determining the player's own priorities, and the short-term and long-term ramifications of that prioritization.

Recall from our basic COI discussion that conflicts do not necessarily imply that the primary interest is truly compromised but rather that circumstances are such that there exists significant risk that the primary interest will be neglected or unduly influenced.[6] It seems sports medicine providers, and especially for those that care for athletes who perform on the biggest and brightest stages, will always be buffeted by steady waves of certain pressures that will compete with the primary interests. It is important for sports medicine providers to recognize that primary and secondary interests may be different among patients and even different for the same patient at different times. As such, each significant treatment decision is a unique process that assimilates relevant medical information in the context of other variables. As mentioned previously, a clinician who has a fairly rigid construct of medicine being only concerned with long-term health will find sports medicine uncomfortable. On the contrary, a clinician who is able to understand a player-patient's drive to perform and achieve now, while balancing, not neglecting, ideals of long-term health, is likely to enjoy the challenges that are ever present in sports medicine at the most competitive levels.

A GAME PLAN

Once, a coach asked a polite but firm question: "what are you going to do to help us win?" That simple request in many ways distilled the essence of the challenges and reality of being a team physician, particularly at the most competitive levels. The author's lofty desire to provide great care to a group of athletes was tempered by reality: the team's goal (and the players making up that team) is to perform, to compete, ... to win. Fortunately, the best interests of the individual frequently line up with the best interests of the team. In other words, what is good for the individual is often good for the team. However, that is not always the case, and this is where the conflicts may arise.

Research into the potential COIs as they relate to pharmaceutical and medical equipment industries suggest it is not enough for the physician to merely be aware of potential for COI.[13] In other words, awareness of the conflict does not necessarily protect the individual in the decision-making process. If this is the case, other strategies need to be created to assist the physician in protecting the decision-making process. The following thoughts represent some observations and ideas based on the author's personal experience and perspective, especially as they pertain to the issues presented previously: confidentiality and clinical decision making.

The author has been extremely fortunate to have worked with organizations that allow the medical staff the freedom to "do right by the patient." When there have been competing interests between the player-patient and team, the medical staff has been supported to err on the side of what is in the best interest of the player. Even in the best of circumstances, it is seemingly inevitable that a team physician will find himself or herself in situations that will be a challenge to the clinician's ability to sort out competing interests and make rational and reasonable decisions.

It is important to define roles and responsibilities on the sports medicine team. Defining expectations and boundaries for the clinician helps identify potential areas of conflict.[2] One example is communication with coaching and administration and this includes the type of information that will be typically discussed for the express purpose of team business and administration. These conversations regarding what health information is appropriate to share are not particularly easy or are likely to be a priority. However, they are important, and for a new team physician or medical staff, should be regarded as critical. Common sense tells us that these topics are best for the off-season, and not during the crucible of a season.

Also with respect to player confidentiality, doctors and athletic trainers should be very familiar with the releases signed by their player-patients that govern the transmission of the content of medical information and to whom. Where possible and practical, a discussion between physician and player regarding the type and flow of player medical information is valuable. Ideally, this exchange could occur at the physical examination. However, this scenario is often not logistically practical. Many team physicians and athletic trainers do have an opportunity to address the team in the preseason, with regard to a number of issues that are germane to the care of the athlete. Perhaps this interaction is the most efficient setting to inform the entire team of this important, and often overlooked, information.

Despite an understanding of the content of the legal documents that guide medical information and confidentiality, the team physician will be confronted with difficult circumstances in which the competing primary interests to the player and to the organization are at odds. With regard to the inevitable "gray" areas, the author has sought to maintain player health information as confidential, unless the condition or issue has become detrimental to performance on or off the field. Alternatively, a condition that places the player-patient, teammates, or competitors at risk will reach the threshold of discussion with team administration. Before this occurs, the need to break confidentiality and discuss the issues with the appropriate limited personnel should be discussed with the player-patient. Even while working in a most favorable team physician environment, it is important for a clinician to have both a healthy self-awareness, and appreciation of particular circumstances and situations that create more risk to the physician and the decision-making process. In other words, all clinicians have vulnerabilities that can affect judgment, and they will vary among individual physicians. A most important antidote to the COIs that exist particularly in professional and collegiate sports is to create appropriate separation from the potential outside influences. Separation may mean minimizing interactions, where practical, with owners/coaches/administration. This may appear odd on the surface, but decreases the chance of being caught in an awkward circumstance in which a conversation about a player may put the physician in an uncomfortable spot. A team physician who develops friendly social relationships with players outside the parameters of the workplace is actually creating circumstances that can have unintended consequences on the physician-patient relationship, especially when difficult and complicated injuries or conditions occur to that player-patient. Long ago, an experienced team physician said "don't read the sports page"; at least as it related to the care of the local team for whom he was caring. This was, and continues to be, very sage advice. This may mean that a physician's exposure to media that pertain to a physician's team/players can have its own subtle effect on a physician's thoughts and perspectives. In this era, insulating oneself from all the various forms of media can be a challenging proposition. The author is not suggesting one must reside in a bunker to make good decisions, but the ubiquitous forms of "the sports page" can have their effect on a professional or major college team physician.

Last, team physicians should be resolute in taking the appropriate time to educate the player-patient as to the ramifications of the different treatment options, both with respect to short-term and long-term effects, as best as can be understood. This physician-patient communication can have enormous influence on the player's decisions. A physician would do well to consistently question himself or herself: am I presenting complete information, and am I presenting it in an unbiased way? Where there is ambiguity in the diagnostic and treatment process, the physician should admit such. Physicians spend countless hours learning how to make correct diagnoses. The most effective team physicians and athletic trainers that the author has been privileged to work with also spend considerable effort on their patient education approach. The best athletic trainers and physicians are also meticulous in the documentation of the nature of these discussions and the outcomes.

SUMMARY

COIs will continue to accompany the role of team physician, particularly at the highest competitive levels. Based on one definition, a COI requires a primary interest, a secondary interest, and a conflict. Two common areas of conflict facing team physicians are confidentiality and clinical decision making.

Confidentiality, a fundamental to the practice of medicine, is altered by the team physician's dual responsibilities to the player-patient and the team. Documents constructed by the team generally specify the parameters by which health information may be handled. Oftentimes, these ground rules are not truly understood by the player or the clinician. Even in the best of circumstances, situations will arise that will challenge the clinician's judgment as to handling of confidential health information. The team doctor should make a strong effort to understand the rules of handling personal health information, and seek to discuss these issues with both the player-patients and team administration in hopes of preempting or minimizing conflicts.

Clinical decision making, classically based on the premise that physicians should promote their patient's long-term health, can be altered by competing interests, including a competitive athlete's goals of short-term personal or team performance, which may be at odds with pursuit of long-term health. There are various positions on the most ethical role of team physicians, but we have evolved primarily to the team physician as the athlete's source of hopefully unbiased clinical information, and assisting the athlete in prioritization of primary and secondary interests. At the same time, team doctors should develop an awareness of the influences on their own decision making, and develop strategies to offset those influences and their ability to distort the pursuit of an athlete's primary interest.

REFERENCES

1. Tucker AM. Ethics and the professional team physician. Clin Sports Med 2004; 23(2):227–41.
2. Holm S, McNamee HJ, Pigozzi F. Ethical practice and sports physician protection: a proposal. Br J Sports Med 2011;45(15):1170–3.
3. Apple D. Team physician-bad ethics, bad business or both? Orthopedics 2002; 25(1):16, 26.
4. Polsky S. Winning medicine: professional sports team doctors' conflict of interest. J Contemp Health Law Policy 1998;14(2):503–29.

5. American College of Sports Medicine. Code of ethics. Available at: http://www. acsm.org/content/navigationmenu/memberservices/memberresources/codeof ethics/Code_of_Ethics.htm. Accessed October 15, 2015.

6. Conflict of interest in medical research, education and practice. Institute of Medicine. In: Lo B, Field MJ, editors. Committee on conflict of interest in medical research, education and practice. Washington, DC: National Academies Press; 2009. p. 44–61.

7. Magee JT, Almekinders LC, Taft TN. HIPAA and the team physician. Sports Medicine Update 2003;4–8.

8. Anderson L. Contractual obligations and the sharing of confidential health information in sport. J Med Ethics 2008;34(9):e6.

9. Baugh CM, Stamm JM, Riley DO, et al. Chronic traumatic encephalopathy: neurodegeneration following repetitive concussive and subconcussive brain trauma. Brain Imaging Behav 2012;6(2):244–54.

10. Goldberg DS. Concussions, professional sports, and conflict of interest: why the National Football League's current policies are bad for its (players') health. HEC Forum 2008;20(4):337–55.

11. Testoni D, Hornik CP, Smith PB, et al. Sports medicine and ethics. Am J Bioeth 2013;13(10):4–12.

12. Bunch WH, Dvonch VM. Informed consent in sports medicine. Clin Sports Med 2004;23(2):183–93.

13. Standaert CJ, Schofferman JA, Herring SA. Expert opinion and controversies in musculoskeletal and sports medicine: conflict of interest. Arch Phys Med Rehabil 2009;90:1647–51.

Ethical Considerations for Analgesic Use in Sports Medicine

Matthew J. Matava, MD*

KEYWORDS

- Ethics • Sports medicine • Analgesics • Injection • Drugs • Medication

KEY POINTS

- Analgesic use in sports medicine includes oral and injectable narcotic and non-narcotic medications as well as local anesthetic agents that may be administered either before, during, or after athletic competition.
- All pain medications given in conjunction with sports activity have the potential to cause both immediate side effects and long-term health consequences that must be considered before use.
- Use of analgesic pain medications in athletes has the potential to exacerbate or worsen the original injury because of the inhibition of the pain response and/or the inflammatory cascade.
- Team physicians must provide full disclosure to the athlete of the most common side effects of analgesic agents used for the purpose of pain management during and after athletic competition. This discussion is optimally held in a controlled setting outside the venue of competitive sports.

INTRODUCTION

No pain, no gain is a common mantra among athletes worldwide in describing their acceptance of pain as a normal consequence of athletic activity. The assumption that in order to gain a competitive advantage, athletes must not only deal with pain but also do whatever they can in order to diminish its effects during competition in order to maximize performance. The general acceptance that exercise and pain often coexist has led to widespread use of both prescription and nonprescription medication before, during, and after exercise and/or athletic competition. In fact, a survey of 563 National Collegiate Athletic Association (NCAA) Division I athletes found that 29% (165) of those surveyed thought there was nothing wrong with using painkillers on the

Disclosure Statement: The author has nothing to disclose.
Department of Orthopedic Surgery, Washington University, St Louis, MO, USA
* 14532 South Outer Forty Drive, Chesterfield, MO 63017.
E-mail address: matavam@wudosis.wustl.edu

day of competition to deal with injury-related pain.[1] Unfortunately, athletes at all levels often do not have the ability to differentiate between activity-related soreness and an actual injury that may be detrimental to both their short-term and long-term health. The team physician must differentiate with which conditions the athlete can safely compete from those that require removal from competition. Players, themselves, may complicate matters by putting pressure on either their personal physicians or their team's medical staff to prescribe or administer analgesics that would allow them to compete. At the collegiate and professional level, an athlete's desire to play may be affected by economic pressures resulting from potential scholarships, lucrative contracts, or the prolongation of their career. The athlete may be tempted to negate the long-term potential health risks for the short-term gain of continued play. As a result, physicians caring for athletes are often faced with the medical and ethical dilemmas of allowing them to compete with injuries and administering pain medication in order to do so.

The purpose of this article is to review the various analgesic agents commonly used by team physicians in an athletic setting, the evidence supporting their use, their most common adverse events in this patient population, and the ethical issues involving pain management in athletes. This review likely does not settle the ethical debate regarding this topic; rather, its purpose is to make physicians and other health care workers who care for athletes aware of the potential consequences and ethical implications of analgesic use in these patients.

NONSTEROIDAL ANTIINFLAMMATORY MEDICATIONS

Beginning with the introduction of ibuprofen in the 1950s, nonsteroidal antiinflammatory drugs (NSAIDs) have been prescribed for mild to moderate muscle and joint pain resulting from athletic injuries or overuse syndromes in an attempt to blunt the body's inflammatory response to injury, control pain, and aid in the return to sports.[2] Because of their popularity in this active patient population, NSAIDs have become the most widely prescribed class of drugs in the world[3] and have been found to be among the most frequently prescribed pharmaceutical in athletes using prescription medication.[4]

Athletes may even take NSAIDs as a preventive measure. For example, during the 2000 Olympic games in Sydney, Canadian athletes used NSAIDs more than any other medication.[5] Tricker[1] found that 29% of 563 collegiate athletes took them to cope with pain on the day of a game. Similarly, Warner and colleagues[6] surveyed 681 high school football players and noted that 452 (75%) used NSAIDs within the past 3 months and one in 7 actually used them daily. Those athletes who used NSAIDs on a daily basis were more likely to perceive improved athletic performance resulting from their use and use them prophylactically without adult supervision. Concerns about inappropriate adolescent use of NSAIDs have been reported. Up to 75% of adolescents use NSAIDs without consulting an adult,[7] and most of these young patients do not recognize the possibility of toxicity from this class of drugs.[8] Unfortunately, these medications are not without complications (see later discussion). Adverse events were reported in 20% of athletes using NSAIDs for a variety of musculoskeletal complaints.[4] Therefore, despite manufacturer warnings against chronic use and their risk of potential complications, it would seem that adolescent athletes are in need of adult supervision as well as education on the appropriate use and potential side effects of this class of drugs.

The antiinflammatory, antipyretic, and analgesic (painkilling) properties of all NSAIDs are mediated through the inhibition of cyclooxygenase (COX), the pivotal enzyme responsible for the conversion of arachidonic acid to prostaglandins and thromboxanes.[9,10] It is now known that there are at least 2 cyclooxygenase subtypes: cyclooxygenase 1 (COX-1) and cyclooxygenase 2 (COX-2). COX-1 is often referred to as a constitutive subtype because it is found in the kidney, gastrointestinal (GI) mucosa, and platelets and results in the maintenance of renal blood flow, production of mucosal and other GI cytoprotective factors, and platelet aggregation. COX-2 is normally found in the brain and kidney and, when induced by inflammatory mediators, becomes measurable in macrophages, gastric epithelium, vascular endothelium, and synoviocytes.

Side Effects of Nonsteroidal Antiinflammatory Drugs

GI symptoms, such as heartburn, nausea, diarrhea, and occult fecal blood loss, are among the most common side effects of NSAIDs and increase in a linear fashion with the daily dose and duration of use.[2,9] These side effects occur via both a systemic mechanism from the inhibition of prostaglandin synthesis as well as through a local irritation of the GI mucosa.

Inhibition of COX activity in the kidney by NSAIDs has relatively mild consequences in healthy individuals but can lead to serious adverse events in patients whose renal function is prostaglandin dependent.[11] Prostaglandin inhibition by NSAIDs may result in sodium retention, hypertension, edema, and hyperkalemia.

NSAIDs may increase the risk of internal bleeding related to their temporary inhibitory effects on platelet function as well as their effects on the GI mucosa.

Cardiovascular toxicity related to nonsalicylated NSAID use is generally not of concern in otherwise healthy young adults. It has been theorized that the disruption in the balance between prostacyclin and thromboxane formation by selective COX-2 inhibitors may increase this risk.[12] In 2005, the Food and Drug Administration (FDA) requested the makers of prescription and over-the-counter nonsalicylated NSAIDs to include a boxed warning highlighting the increased risk for cardiovascular events as well as GI toxicity, including the risk for life-threatening GI bleeding.

Studies have also shown that various NSAIDs may impair bone healing because of their inhibitory affect on prostaglandins, which are vital for the formation of osteoclastic and osteoblastic precursor cells. Several animal and human clinical trials suggest that NSAIDs negatively impact fracture healing.[13] However, no study has linked ketorolac use to delayed healing of athletically induced stress fractures.

Systemic side effects to the use of NSAIDs include headache, vasodilatation, asthma, and weight gain related to fluid retention, all of which might negatively affect athletic performance in the short term.

Ketorolac Tromethamine (Toradol)

Ketorolac tromethamine (Toradol) is a nonspecific COX inhibitor and as such inhibits both isoforms of COX decreasing synthesis of prostaglandins. It has potent analgesic and antiinflammatory properties that can be administered orally, intravenously (IV), intramuscularly (IM), and intranasally. Ketorolac has been used principally for its analgesic properties following acute strains and sprains, overuse injuries, and as an adjunct to narcotic medication following surgery. In addition to the antiinflammatory effects of ketorolac, its effect to decrease prostaglandin levels, which decreases the sensitivity of afferent nerve receptors, thereby, ameliorating pain.[14] Several studies have shown ketorolac to be as effective and, in some cases, more effective than opioids for pain control in various dental pain models, pain conditions, and following anterior cruciate ligament reconstruction.[15–17] It is unknown whether there are different dose-response relationships between analgesic and antiinflammatory effects.

Ketorolac reaches its peak plasma concentration within 20 minutes when taken orally and within 45 minutes when administered via an IM route.[18] The elimination half-life and renal clearance are similar between oral and IM administration, though time to maximum concentration has been shown to be only 20 minutes for oral ketorolac compared with 45 minutes for the IM route.[18] Jung and colleagues[19] compared a single 10-mg dose of ketorolac via IV, IM, and oral routes to 15 healthy subjects. They found that the mean plasma concentration-time curves for all 3 routes were nearly identical. Given this pharmacokinetic profile, the oral and IM dose equivalents are theoretically the same such that an oral dose of 30 mg has the same drug kinetics as an IM dose of 30 mg except that the oral route has approximately a 30-minute earlier peak concentration and presumably time of peak effect.[18] Oral ketorolac was originally evaluated and approved by the FDA only after IM or IV administration. However, the drug is now most commonly given alone in its oral form, which would be considered an off-label usage, which should be considered when given to an athlete. This topic must be addressed with the athlete before use.

Ketorolac is indicated for the short-term (up to 5 days in adults) management of moderately severe acute pain that requires analgesia at the opioid level and only as continuation treatment following IV or IM dosing of ketorolac, if necessary.[20] Because ketorolac inhibits platelet function it is, therefore, contraindicated in patients with hemorrhagic diathesis, incomplete hemostasis, and those at high risk of bleeding.[21–24] Despite the theoretic association between ketorolac and the risk of hemorrhage, there have been no studies documenting a bleeding complication related to its use following contact or collision sports. Mynster and Singer[25] investigated the effects of IM ketorolac on the bleeding times of 20 healthy volunteers. The investigators found that a single 60-mg injection of ketorolac was associated with a 50% prolongation of the bleeding time 4 hours following injection, but they were unable to determine if this finding was clinically relevant.[25] Tokish and colleagues[26] commented that this effect warrants reconsideration of game-day injections for National Football League (NFL) players.

Issues Associated with Sports-Related Nonsteroidal Antiinflammatory Drug Use

Both prescription and over-the-counter NSAIDs have been used extensively to treat various musculoskeletal injuries. Unfortunately, the inflammatory cascade that naturally occurs following a muscle, tendon, ligament, or bone injury may be inhibited by these drugs because of their affect on inflammation. Without the normal inflammatory cascade, natural tissue healing could be delayed or even inhibited.

Studies have shown an NSAID-associated delay in healing of tibial fractures, humeral shaft fractures, and other various long-bone fractures; however, most of the published studies in humans are retrospective in design.[13] Indomethacin, widely used to inhibit heterotopic ossification, was found to be associated with a 29% rate of long-bone fracture nonunion compared with 7% seen with placebo and radiation therapy.[27] Therefore, despite the differences in patient populations between athletes and those treated in the studies referenced earlier, physicians caring for athletes who sustain fractures should at least discuss the risk of delayed fracture healing associated with NSAID use. From these findings, avoidance of NSAIDs in the setting of acute traumatic fractures or stress fractures at higher risk for nonunion is recommended,[13] as the potential diminution in postinjury pain may not be worth the increased risk of impaired fracture healing.

Ketorolac injections have been used for several years in the NFL and more recently in Major League Baseball and the NCAA to treat musculoskeletal injuries and to prevent postgame soreness. The only study, to date, examining the prevalence of ketorolac use in professional sports was performed by Tokish and colleagues[26] in 2002.

These researchers investigated the use of injectable ketorolac in NFL teams during the 2001 season. Their study revealed that 28 of the 30 teams that responded to their survey used IM ketorolac. Game-day usage was reported at 93%, with pain relief of 1 to 2 days noted in 50% to 75% of players. There were 6 adverse reactions reported, including 4 muscle injuries, one GI complaint, and one case of postinjection soreness. Anecdotally, some NFL medical staffs were of the opinion that their players thought that "getting a shot" was an "intrinsic sign" that they were getting a more powerful medicine.[26] Overall, these researchers found ketorolac to be safe and effective when used in the pregame setting of the NFL.

Injections are typically perceived as a more aggressive form of treatment that has recently garnered attention from the lay media as a result of ketorolac injections used before competition in the NFL and NCAA Division I football.[28,29] Injection of medication to treat sports-related conditions is not unheard of, but there is no evidence of increased effectiveness from this route of administration. Public perception of team physicians administering various therapeutic (or painkilling) injections to allow athletes to return to competition likely varies depending on the level of competition and public visibility of the athlete. Moreover, the literature is deficient in terms of the ethical considerations implicit with the administration of injectable medications (as opposed to oral medications) in the athletic setting solely in order for the athlete to return to competition. Any discussion of the ethical implications of a medical treatment must take into consideration the rational use of the drug or therapy in the context in which it is administered.

In general, professional and collegiate athletes are superbly fit and healthy with little risk of experiencing any of the known complications associated with the use of ketorolac. However, given the nature of American football and the risk of injury associated with other collision sports, the NFL Physicians Society assembled a Toradol Task Force to provide NFL physicians with therapeutic *guidelines* on the use of ketorolac in order to decrease the potential risk of hemorrhage resulting from a significant collision or trauma. Thus far, there have been no documented cases of severe complications associated with the use of ketorolac in NFL players. However, one Division I collegiate football player has publicly attributed his myocardial infarction to repeated game-day injections over the course of a season. The Toradol Task Force was also concerned with the perceived increase in NFL players requesting IM ketorolac injections as a *prophylactic* medication in order to reduce the anticipated pain during as well as after competition. The perception of NFL players getting shot up before competition has shed an unfavorable light on the NFL as well as on team physicians who are perceived as being complicit with the players' desire to play at all costs, irrespective of the medical consequences. Finally, given their relative safety, proven efficacy, and similar pharmacokinetic profiles of oral ketorolac compared with the IM route of administration, it would seem preferable to use the lowest oral dose of ketorolac instead of the IM or IV forms. The fact that oral ketorolac has a quicker onset of action than the IM form also favors the oral route of administration. Because ketorolac's bioavailability depends on plasma volume rather than body mass, the same dose can be administered to a 300-lb lineman as would be given to a 200-lb wide receiver.

As a result of the before mentioned issues, the NFL Physician Society Toradol Task Force published the following recommendations in 2012 for ketorolac use in the NFL acknowledging that each team physician is ultimately free to practice medicine as he or she feels is in the best interest of patients within the standard of care.[30] These proposed recommendations were based on the available evidence taking into consideration the pharmacokinetic properties of ketorolac's multiple formulations, its accepted indications and contraindications, and the unique clinical challenges of the NFL. It was thought that these recommendations would not only reduce the potential occurrence of side effects but also maintain competitive balance taking into consideration the perceived, yet unproven, psychological benefits associated with the use of ketorolac.

National Football League Team Physician Society Toradol Task Force Recommendations

- Ketorolac should only be administered under the direct supervision and order of a team physician.[30]
- Ketorolac should not be used prophylactically as a means of reducing anticipated pain either during or after participation in NFL games or practices.[29]
- Ketorolac use should be limited to those players diagnosed with an injury or condition and listed on the teams' latest injury report or following a physician-diagnosed injury or condition that occurs after the last injury report has been submitted to the NFL before competition.[29]
- Ketorolac should be given in the lowest effective therapeutic dose and should not be used in any form for more than 5 days. There is no evidence that an increase in dosage is necessary for players with larger body mass.[29]
- Ketorolac should be given in its oral preparation under typical circumstances as it is recognized that the oral preparation (1) has a faster onset of action than the IM preparation, (2) has a duration of action that is equivalent to the IM and IV forms, and (3) has a plasma concentration-time curve that is nearly identical to the IM and IV preparations.[29]
- IM and IV injection of ketorolac should not be used except *following* an acute, game-related injury whereby significant visceral or central nervous system (CNS) bleeding is not expected and other oral or intranasal pain medications are inadequate or not tolerated. If IM or IV ketorolac is thought to be appropriate by the treating physician, the lowest possible dosage should be used.[29]
- Ketorolac should not be taken concurrently with other NSAIDs.[29]
- Ketorolac should not be taken by those players with a history of allergic reaction to ketorolac, other NSAIDs, or aspirin. In addition, a player with a history of significant GI bleeding, renal compromise, or a past history of complications related to NSAIDs should not take ketorolac.[29]

NARCOTIC ANALGESICS

The nature of athletic competition, especially in those sports involving frequent contact or collision, would suggest that the risk of significant musculoskeletal injury is a very real possibility. As a result, team physicians must occasionally rely on narcotic pain medications to control the acute pain following the injury, irrespective of the need for surgery. Narcotic pain medications are considered any class of substances that blunt the senses; that in large quantities produce euphoria, stupor, or coma; that when used constantly can cause habituation or addiction; and that are used in medicine to relieve pain, cause sedation, and induce sleep.[31,32] Narcotic pain medications work by binding to one of 3 types of opioid receptors, mu (μ), delta (δ), and kappa (κ), which are present in the central and peripheral nervous system.[33] These receptors facilitate opening of potassium channels (causing hyperpolarization) or inhibit calcium channel opening, which inhibits release of excitatory neurotransmitters, such as substance P, to reduce neuronal excitability in the pain-carrying pathway.[34] When these drugs attach to their receptors, they reduce the perception of pain and can produce a sense of well-being analogous to when they are activated by the body's own endogenous opioid chemicals (endorphins, encephalins).[35]

Side Effects of Narcotic Analgesics

Common side effects of narcotic analgesic medications include sedation, dizziness, nausea, vomiting, constipation, respiratory depression, physical dependence, and tolerance, with the most being constipation and nausea.[36] Physical dependence and tolerance may occur, as larger doses are required to achieve the same degree of analgesic effect. Physical dependence ensues following several weeks of continued use and may result in withdrawal symptoms, such as muscle pain, irritability, anxiety, nausea, diarrhea, and vomiting. Ultimately, with long-standing use, addiction can develop as a neurobiological disease characterized by one or more of the following behaviors: impaired control over drug use, compulsive use, continued use despite harm, and craving.[35]

Regulation of Narcotic Medication

Narcotic medications are considered controlled substances by the Drug Enforcement Agency (DEA). Drugs and other substances that are classified as controlled substances under the Controlled Substances Act (CSA) are divided into 5 schedules (**Table 1**).[31,37] Substances are placed in their respective schedules based on whether they have a currently accepted medical use in the United States, their relative abuse potential, and likelihood of causing dependence when abused.

Tramadol (Ultram)

Tramadol (Ultram) is an opiate pain medication used to treat moderate to severe pain resulting from acute and chronic injuries or conditions. The onset of action is usually within an hour and peaks within 2 to 4 hours. Tramadol has 2 different mechanisms of action: (1) binding to the μ-opioid receptor and (2) inhibition of serotonin and norepinephrine reuptake.[38] On a dose-by-dose basis, tramadol has approximately one-tenth the potency of morphine. The side effect profile of tramadol is similar to other narcotic analgesics.

Tramadol was originally released in 1995 as an opiate agonist and not a narcotic. As a result, it was not monitored as a controlled substance by the DEA and could be prescribed, distributed, and stored similar to any other noncontrolled pain medication. Team physicians used tramadol as a useful adjunct in the sports medicine setting when an athlete required medication instead of or in addition to NSAIDs for acute pain. However, given the addictive nature of similar opioid analgesics, the high potential for tramadol's nonmedical misuse, and its ease of illegal distribution, tramadol was placed into schedule IV of the federal CSA on August 14, 2014.[39] This change was met with significant debate. The author is unaware of any clinical reports of an athlete suffering a significant complication as a result of tramadol use in an athletic setting. Nevertheless, team physicians are no longer able to freely prescribe, store, or administer tramadol for reasons similar to other controlled substances.

Increasing Use and Abuse of Narcotic Medication

Chronic pain conditions and prescription drug abuse are becoming important public health issues. Population-based studies reveal that more than 75 million Americans (about 25% of the entire population) have chronic or recurrent pain. Of these, 40% report the pain as having a moderate to severe impact on their lives.[40] As a result, the number of prescriptions for narcotic medications have escalated from approximately 76 million in 1991 to nearly 207 million in 2013, with the United States the

Table 1
Definition of controlled substance schedules

Schedule I controlled substances	Substances in this schedule have no currently accepted medical use in the United States, a lack of accepted safety for use under medical supervision, and a high potential for abuse.	Examples: heroin, lysergic acid diethylamide, marijuana, 3,4-methylenedioxymethamphetamine (ecstasy), methaqualone, and peyote
Schedule II controlled substances	Substances in this schedule have a high potential for abuse, which may lead to severe psychological or physical dependence.	Examples: hydromorphone (Dilaudid), methadone (Dolophine), meperidine (Demerol), oxycodone (OxyContin, Percocet), and fentanyl (Duragesic); other schedule II narcotics: morphine, opium, codeine, and hydrocodone
Schedule III controlled substances	Substances in this schedule have a potential for abuse less than substances in schedules I or II, and abuse may lead to moderate or low physical dependence or high psychological dependence.	Examples: products containing not more than 90 mg of codeine per dosage unit (Tylenol with Codeine)
Schedule IV controlled substances	Substances in this schedule have a low potential for abuse relative to substances in schedule III.	Examples: alprazolam (Xanax), carisoprodol (Soma), clonazepam (Klonopin), clorazepate (Tranxene), diazepam (Valium), lorazepam (Ativan), midazolam (Versed), temazepam (Restoril), and triazolam (Halcion)
Schedule V controlled substances	Substances in this schedule have a low potential for abuse relative to substances listed in schedule IV and consist primarily of preparations containing limited quantities of certain narcotics.	Examples: cough preparations containing not more than 200 mg of codeine per 100 mL or per 100 g (Robitussin AC, Phenergan with Codeine), and ezogabine

From Controlled substance schedules. Resources. US Department of Justice. Available at: http://www.deadiversion.usdoj.gov/schedules/index.html#define. Accessed August 2, 2015.

largest consumer globally, accounting for almost 100% of the world consumption of hydrocodone (eg, Vicodin) and 81% of oxycodone (eg, Percocet).[41] There were an estimated 2.1 million people in the United States with substance-use disorders related to prescription opioid pain relievers in 2012, and the number of unintentional overdose deaths from prescription pain relievers has more than quadrupled since 1999.[42] These statistics include, in part, drastic increases in the number of narcotic prescriptions written and dispensed, greater social acceptance for using medications to relieve physical and mental pain, and aggressive marketing by pharmaceutical companies. These factors together have helped create the broad "environmental availability" of prescription medications in general and narcotic analgesics in particular.[35]

Unintended Consequences of Narcotic Use in Athletes

No one would question the use of these drugs in the controlled environment of a hospital or other health care facility where the injury is definitively evaluated and treated. However, the use of narcotics as a means to allow an immediate return to play following an injury has received increased scrutiny. A survey by Cotler and colleagues[43] found that 52% of 644 retired NFL players with an average playing career of 7.6 years admitted to using prescription pain medication during their playing days. Of those, 71% admitted to misusing the drugs then, and 15% of the misusers admitted to misusing the medication within the past 30 days. Interestingly, 63% of those surveyed who used narcotic pain pills while playing obtained the medications from a nonmedical source, such as a teammate, coach, trainer, relative, dealer, or the Internet. Reports in the popular media[29] suggest that NFL athletes are at an increased risk for abuse of prescription painkillers as a result of the frequent rate of injury in football, a pervasive culture of playing with pain, indiscriminate administration of pain medication by medical personnel, rampant narcotic overconsumption in the general population, and the absence of standardized league-wide monitoring. Anecdotal reports of opioid use in amateur athletes in order to return to play also exist in the lay media.[44] In one of the few studies on the subject, Darrow and colleagues[45] found that adolescents who participated in high-risk sports, such as football or wrestling, had a 50% greater risk of nonmedical use of prescription narcotics than adolescents who did not participate in these types of sports. It may be surmised that these greater odds may be related to the fact that football and wrestling have the highest severe injury rate among high school athletes or that these athletes may have an increased opportunity to get opioids from a teammate who may be diverting opioid medication to his peers.[46]

Most would agree that the practice of medicine is an art influenced by science and that the standard of care for many medical conditions is silent on the use of pain medication in conjunction with definitive treatment. The culture of pain medication use in professional sports, such as football, has evolved over the past several years to become less acceptable than in prior decades. The reasons for this change are multifactorial and can be attributed, in part, to more restrictive federal regulations, tightened physician prescribing practices, enhanced awareness of the incidence and consequences of narcotic addiction in the United States, increased scrutiny by the lay media, and greater recognition by risk-averse athletic governing bodies. Easterbrook[29] has suggested that a league such as the NFL could publicize anonymous data on drug-prescribing practices of its team physicians or prohibit players from returning to the field less than 24 hours after receiving a prescription pain medication in order to enhance player safety even further. Such practices would be arbitrary and would require joint acceptance by both the governing league and the Player's Association, which would be highly unlikely.

A team physician is ultimately free to dispense painkillers as he or she sees fit within the framework of the clinical condition, prudent judgment, and the context in which the injury took place. Physicians are limited by their DEA license to only prescribe, administer, or distribute controlled narcotic substances within the state in which they are licensed to practice medicine. In addition, the practical aspects of secure drug storage and the mounting regulatory hurdles that clinicians must face in order store or distribute controlled substances make the routine availability of these drugs to athletes at an athletic venue very difficult. Aside from the ethical aspects of administering narcotics in order to return a player to competition, there exist severe legal ramifications for physicians who prescribe or distribute narcotic medications to their athletes outside of their state of licensure, irrespective of the medical indication. Many team physicians have had little specific training in the use of pain medication and addiction medicine and, therefore, may lack the foundation on which to safely base their prescribing patterns in this patient population. In addition, the high prevalence of psychiatric comorbidity in those who misuse or abuse prescription drugs contributes to the complexity of this issue.

There would seem to be no valid medical or ethical indication to prescribe a narcotic pain medication to an adolescent or amateur athlete in order to return to play following an acute injury. If the athlete has been definitively treated for the orthopedic condition but his or her pain level requires narcotic-strength medication, then return to sports should likely not be considered. Professional athletes often face other, more tangible, nonmedical issues, such as performance bonuses, contract extensions, or end-of-career decisions, that may strongly influence their desire to use narcotic pain medication either openly or through more clandestine means. Although the occasional use of a single narcotic tablet in an otherwise healthy 320-lb lineman may not lead to a life of addiction and illicit drug use, its use should not be trivialized considering the potential immediate effects of impaired mentation or judgment that may result in a more devastating injury. The tenant, *primum non nocere* (first do no harm) must always be respected.

INJECTABLE ANESTHETICS USED IN SPORTS

Injectable local anesthetic agents have been used in the United States since the 1960s in the treatment of athletes injured during competition. Anesthetic use in suturing an acute laceration is not considered for the purposes of this discussion. In addition, a review of corticosteroid injections used to reduce inflammation as a treatment modality for various musculoskeletal conditions is beyond the scope of this article. Rather, the emphasis here is on the use of local analgesics injected directly into the site of a musculoskeletal injury for the intended purpose of providing *immediate* temporary pain relief so that the athlete can resume play.

There is a paucity of information in the published sports medicine literature regarding the use of local anesthetic agents in athletes.[47,48] A reason for this seems to be the pervasive opinion that the practice of administering analgesic injections in athletes is considered unethical by some practitioners and governing organizations despite an absence of evidence-based conclusions to dispel this practice. For example, the International Rugby Board, which administers the sport of Rugby Union, has officially banned local anesthetic use for painkilling purposes. In addition, the International Federation of Sports Medicine (FIMS) based in Lausanne, Switzerland to promote and advance the practice of sports medicine worldwide has issued a policy that states that: "[The physician may not]… in any way mask pain in order to enable the athlete's return to practicing the sport if there is any risk of aggravating the injury."[49] However, the "NCAA Sports Medicine Handbook" leaves local injections to the discretion of the treating physician "since there is little scientific research on the subject."[50] Most of the published literature on this subject deals primarily with case reports of complications resulting from either systemic toxicity from the anesthetic agent or their inadvertent injection into tissues other than the intended area of injury.

Local anesthetic agents can only be reasonably expected to work for an injury localized to a specific site, such as an individual joint or discreet soft tissue location easily identified by an area of point tenderness. Diffuse regions of discomfort (ie, quadriceps strain) are not effectively anesthetized because the volume of anesthetic agent required would be impractical, ineffective, and unsafe from a toxicity standpoint. In addition, large weight-bearing joints (ie, knee, ankle) are not to be injected because the loss of pain sensation and proprioception would be detrimental to the health of the joint. Regional blockades commonly used in the postoperative management of pain are also contraindicated because the resulting diffuse muscle paralysis, loss of protective sensation, and absence of position sense would put the athlete at significant risk for further injury in addition to precluding any type of athletic activity.

Typical agents used are 1% or 2% lidocaine (Xylocaine), 0.25% or 0.5% bupivacaine (Marcaine), and 3% mepivacaine (Carbocaine). Some practitioners prefer to use an anesthetic combined with epinephrine in order to cause vasoconstriction of the injected area in order to lengthen the duration of activity. The use of these drugs in combination with epinephrine or other vasoconstrictive agents in the fingers, toes, earlobes and other areas where a decrease in circulation, even if only temporary, could result in significant harm. The volume of injected anesthetic depends on the size of the intended area; however, the treating physician should be familiar with the maximum allowable doses of the drug used based on the patients' body weight.

The local skin overlying the intended area to be injected should always be prepped in a sterile fashion with povidone-iodine (Betadine), chlorhexidine, or alcohol in order to reduce the rare but present risk of deep or superficial infection. Sterile preparation may reduce the risk of infection, but this can be challenging in the game-day training room or hotel setting. In addition, injections clearly pose a risk of bleeding and injury to adjacent structures. The athlete should be apprised that these analgesics are short-lived, nontherapeutic, and risk further damage to the injured area. As with the administration of any other form of invasive treatment, informed consent has been recommended before administering injections to athletes[48]; the procedure should also be documented as in any clinical encounter. Most high school athletes are too young to legally provide consent; thus, parents must be consulted if injections are considered as a part of the pain management plan. However, it can be strongly argued that anesthetic injections used to allow a high school athlete to return to play is impractical, overly aggressive, and likely not indicated.

These agents typically take effect within 5 minutes, which is advantageous to a rapid return to competition. The degree and duration of pain relief depends on the size, depth, and degree of injury as well as on the agent used. Bupivacaine typically has the longest duration of action (2 to 6 hours), though this time may be decreased by the increased blood flow to the injected area seen in athletic activity. Typically, an athlete only requires 2 to 3 hours of pain control to complete competition, as these drugs are not expected to provide lasting pain relief. There is no role for the concurrent administration of corticosteroid medications at the same time the local anesthetic is given in an athletic setting.

Local anesthetic agents are contraindicated for any history of hypersensitivity reactions to the individual agents or to amino-amide anesthetics. Fortunately, allergic reactions are rare. Athletes typically will not have any history or knowledge of an allergy to these drugs, though this should be addressed before injection. Adverse drugs reactions (ADRs) to local anesthetics are rare when they are administered correctly. Most ADRs are caused by accelerated absorption from the injection site, unintentional intravascular injection, or slow metabolic degradation. Clinically significant adverse events result from systemic absorption of the drug and primarily involve the CNS and cardiovascular system. At higher plasma concentrations, both inhibitory and excitatory pathways are inhibited, causing CNS depression and potentially coma. Other CNS side effects include perioral numbness, facial tingling, vertigo, tinnitus, dizziness, and seizure. Cardiovascular side effects include hypotension, arrhythmia, bradycardia, heart block, and cardiac arrest. Compared with other local anesthetics, bupivacaine is markedly cardiotoxic. Other less common side effects include bronchospasm, dyspnea, respiratory depression or arrest, metallic taste, nausea, vomiting, and tinnitus.

Orchard[49] published the largest series of local anesthetic agents in professional athletes. He retrospectively reviewed his experience over a 6-year period in the use of local anesthetic agents for 3 rugby and Australian-rules football teams. There were 268 injuries for which local anesthetic was used to allow early return to play. He noted 11 minor (degenerative arthritis of a small joint, inadvertent sensory loss, failure of the injection) and 6 major (fracture, ligament rupture, tendon rupture, inadvertent motor block) complications, although none of these were catastrophic or career ending. Interestingly, approximately 10% of players on these 3 teams required the use of a local anesthetic in order to compete. Injuries in which he thought the reward of an injection outweighed the risk included acromioclavicular joint sprain, phalangeal injuries of fingers/toes 2 through 5, rib and sternum injuries (unspecified), iliac crest contusion, and chronic plantar fasciitis. Injuries in which the risk outweighed the benefit included ankle sprains, tendon injuries, prepatellar and olecranon bursitis, and first metacarpal and radiocarpal injuries. He provided no opinion as to the safety of injecting large, weight-bearing joints. He concluded that the use of local anesthetic in professional rugby may reduce the rates of players missing matches through injury; but there is the risk of worsening the injury, which should be fully explained to players. A procedure should only be used when both the doctor and player consider that the benefits outweigh the risks. What constitutes a safe injection likely depends on the individual athlete, his or her comfort level with an injection, and the personal opinion and experience level of the team physician.

It must be recognized that multiple examples of complications exist both in the short-term as well as following the repetitive injection of anesthetics into an injured area. For example, in 2002, an NFL running back, Jerome Bettis, was forced to leave a game because of an inadvertent femoral block following a local injection for a groin strain. Another NFL player, Mark Siani, reportedly received a weekly injection for 16 weeks into a broken toe. In several of these cases, the team physicians were successfully sued following allegations of negligence related to the injection of a local anesthetic agent that purportedly caused a premature degeneration of the involved area resulting in the athlete's forced retirement.[51] In several such cases, it is difficult to determine whether the ensuing deterioration in the involved area was caused by the injection that allowed the athlete to do further damage or the natural history of the original injury.

In the absence of objective evidence to help guide decision making, physicians are faced with the dilemma of complying with the wishes of the player who typically will do whatever it takes to return to play and the potential for exacerbating an injury. Medicine, in general, has evolved from a paternalistic approach whereby the physician does what he or she feels is best for patients irrespective of their opinion or unique set of circumstances to that of shared decision making. In this situation, it would seem that a middle ground would be most appropriate whereby the physician counsels patients regarding the efficacy, contraindications, side effects, and long-term risks of anesthetic injections while respecting the athletes' wishes, yet still maintaining responsibility to prevent the athletes from making careless decisions in the heat of competition.

In order to avoid all potential risk of exacerbating an injury or the premature onset of degenerative joint disease, some governing bodies have outlawed all anesthetic injections. However, this edict is impractical and likely unenforceable. Even if a team physician is prevented from using an anesthetic injection for a dislocated finger, is he or she also prevented from using a local anesthetic injection to suture a laceration? Is the risk for permanent injury greater if an acromioclavicular joint is injected or an athlete with known osteoarthritis of the knee with an associated meniscal tear is allowed to

Table 2
Options for athletic administrative bodies regarding local anesthetic policy

Option	Banning of All Local Anesthetic Use	Legal with Compulsory Notification of All Use	No Regulation
Sports and governing bodies with this approach	Rugby Union FIMS	Olympic soccer competition (in theory)	American football, most soccer competitions, Australian-rules football, rugby league, NCAA
Advantages	It would result in reduced use of local anesthetic injection for painkilling purposes, lessening any complications. From a medicolegal basis, it would absolve governing body administrators from liability.	The incidence and complications of local anesthetic use could be monitored. If combined with a comprehensive surveillance system, long-term follow-up regarding the safety of anesthetic agents could be obtained.	Administrators transfer much of their liability over to the treating doctor. The decision whether to use a local anesthetic is made between doctor and patients only.
Disadvantages	Exceptions must be made to the basic rule (eg, suturing of lacerations), and it is almost impossible to draw a fair line for the exceptions. Such a law would be almost impossible to police, which would make it tempting and easy for certain players to violate, creating a paradox whereby cheats were not caught and so those obeying the rules were disadvantaged. Players may unnecessarily miss important games in cases when local anesthetic use would be safe.	It is costly to administer because it should be combined with a comprehensive injury surveillance system and a drug testing program to be effective. It is difficult to achieve full compliance. By having a notification process, the extent of local anesthetic use becomes known, which may initially increase the medicolegal liability for administrative bodies.	Other than the tort law system, there is very little regulation of possible misuse of this technique. Because the use remains a private matter, there is little opportunity to research the short- and long-term complications of these techniques.
Conclusion	It is impractical and creates a terrible dilemma for doctors and players working in such an environment.	It is probably the best option for professional sports in the future.	It allows the status quo (lack of evidence-based guidelines to base medical recommendations), which is undesirable.

Adapted from Orchard J. Is it safe to use local anesthetic painkilling injections in professional football. Sports Med 2004;34:214; with permission.

compete in the absence of symptoms? In the absence of scientific evidence, it would seem that those governing bodies that have outlawed anesthetic injections in the competitive setting are merely shielding themselves from liability by transferring it to the team physician. A tenable solution to this would be a compulsory league-wide registry whereby the governing body administrators, players' union, and team physician group work in unison to document the incidence, context, and complications of these injections so that reliable data could be generated in a relatively rapid fashion to guide the practice without generating increased medicolegal liability for the physicians. Orchard[51] has listed the relevant advantages and disadvantages of the various approaches to a league-wide policy on anesthetic agents with the practical conclusion likely to occur for each approach (**Table 2**).

In summary, the use of local anesthetic injections in the athletic setting seems to be relatively widespread at both the collegiate and professional level. There is no published literature or opinion regarding their use at the high school level, though the absence of routine physician coverage and the unavailability of medical supplies at high school sports venues likely present practical impediments for their use in these athletes. The injection of a local anesthetic agent in an athletic setting should only be administered by a qualified clinician who is licensed to perform this procedure and who is familiar with the drug's actions and adverse effects as well as the local anatomy. The treating clinician should be well aware of the quantity of these agents that can be safely injected based on the athlete's body weight. These agents should only be administered in facilities equipped to handle any allergic reaction, including a cardiopulmonary emergency, which may follow their use. Anesthetic injections should only be administered when medically justified, when the risk of administration is fully explained to patients, when the use is not harmful to continued athletic activity, and when they will not jeopardize the ability of the athlete to protect himself or herself from either aggravating the preexisting injury or cause further injury to another body part. This factor is most relevant to the debate surrounding their use.

SUMMARY

Team physicians who care for high-level athletes at both the amateur and professional levels are often faced with the challenge of administering analgesic medications during a competitive setting or in order to allow an athlete to return to play or training. A variety of analgesics are available to the clinician, all with differing mechanisms of action, efficacy, short-term side effects, and long-term risks to the athlete's general health. The treating physician must also balance the risk of the analgesic actually causing the athlete to either delay the time to complete healing or cause an exacerbation of the original injury because of an inhibition of the pain response. The potential increased risk of administering pain medication in a competitive athletic setting is difficult to quantify separately from the natural history of the original injury. Unfortunately, the available studies dealing with this topic are often flawed in design, nonrandomized, lacking a control group, or underpowered to provide meaningful evidence-based recommendations for the clinician. As in other areas of orthopedic sports medicine, the treating physician must ultimately integrate the available research with experience, good judgment, and the individual circumstances affecting each athlete to formulate a treatment plan that involves analgesic use in the athletic setting.

REFERENCES

1. Tricker R. Painkilling drugs in collegiate athletics. J Drug Educ 2000;30:313–24.

2. Shoor S. Athletes, nonsteroidal anti-inflammatory drugs, coxibs, and the gastro-intestinal tract. Curr Sports Med Rep 2002;1:107–15.
3. Baum C, Kennedy DL, Forbes MB. Utilization of nonsteroidal anti-inflammatory drugs. Arthritis Rheum 1985;28:686–92.
4. Alaranta A, Alaranta H, Helenius I. Use of prescription drugs in athletes. Sports Med 2008;38(6):449–63.
5. Lippi G, Franchini M, Guidi GC. Non steroidal anti-inflammatory drugs (NSAIDs) in athletes. Br J Sports Med 2006;40:661–3.
6. Warner DC, Schnepf G, Barret MS, et al. Prevalence, attitudes and behaviors related to the use of nonsteroidal anti-inflammatory drugs (NSAIDs) in student athletes. J Adolesc Health 2002;30:150–3.
7. Chambers CT, Reid GJ, McGrath PJ, et al. Self-administration of over-the-counter medication for pain among adolescents. Arch Pediatr Adolesc Med 1997;151: 449–55.
8. Huott M, Storrow A. A survey of adolescents' knowledge regarding toxicity of over-the-counter medications. Acad Emerg Med 1997;4:214–8.
9. Feucht CL, Patel DR. Analgesics and anti-inflammatory medications in sports - use and abuse. Pediatr Clin North Am 2010;57:751–74.
10. Ziltener JL, Leal S, Fournier PE. Non-steroidal anti-inflammatory drugs for athletes - an update. Ann Phys Rehabil Med 2010;53:278–88.
11. Brater DC. Anti-inflammatory agents and renal function. Semin Arthritis Rheum 2002;32(3):33–42.
12. American College of Rheumatology Ad Hoc Group on Use of Selective and Non-selective Nonsteroidal Anti-inflammatory Drugs. Recommendations for use of selective and nonselective nonsteroidal anti-inflammatory drugs - an American College of Rheumatology white paper. Arthritis Rheum 2008;59(8): 1058–73.
13. Mehallo CJ, Drezner JA, Bytomski JR. Practical management: nonsteroidal anti-inflammatory drug (NSAID) use in athletic injuries. Clin J Sport Med 2006;16(2): 170–4.
14. Dietzel DP, Hedlund EC. Injections and return to play. Curr Sports Med Rep 2004; 3:310–5.
15. Barber FA, Gladu DE. Comparison of oral ketorolac and hydrocodone for pain relief after anterior cruciate ligament reconstruction. Arthroscopy 1998;14: 605–12.
16. McGuire DA, Sanders K, Hendricks SD. Comparison of ketorolac and opioid analgesics in postoperative ACL reconstruction outpatient pain control. Arthros-copy 1993;9:653–61.
17. Milne JC, Russell JA, Woods GW, et al. Effect of ketorolac tromethamine (Toradol) on Ecchymosis following anterior cruciate ligament reconstruction. Am J Knee Surg 1995;1:24–7.
18. Buckley MMT, Brogden RN. Ketorolac - a review of its pharmacodynamic and pharmacokinetic properties, and therapeutic potential. Drugs 1990;39:86–109.
19. Jung D, Mroszczak E, Bynum L. Pharmacokinetics of ketorolac tromethamine in humans after intravenous, intramuscular, and oral administration. Eur J Pharma-col 1988;35:423–5.
20. Ketorolac Tromethamine. PDR.Net. PDR. Available at: http://www.pdr.net/drug-summary/Ketorolac-Tromethamine-Tablets-ketorolac-tromethamine-1793.3935. Accessed August 2, 2015.
21. Concannon MJ, Meng L, Welsh CF, et al. Inhibition of perioperative platelet aggre-gation using Toradol (Ketorolac). Ann Plast Surg 1993;3:264–6.

22. Fragen RJ, Stulberg SD, Wixson R, et al. Effect of ketorolac tromethamine on bleeding and on requirements for analgesia after total knee arthroplasty. J Bone Joint Surg Am 1995;77-A:998–1002.

23. Strom BL, Berlin JA, Kinman JL, et al. Parenteral ketorolac and risk of gastrointestinal and operative site bleeding: a postmarketing surveillance study. JAMA 1996; 275:376–82.

24. Niemi TT, Taxell C, Rosenberg PH. Comparison of intravenous ketoprofen, ketorolac, and diclofenac on platelet function in volunteers. Acta Anaesthesiol Scand 1997;41:1353–8.

25. Mynster CI, Singer AJ. Effect of intramuscular Toradol on bleeding times [abstract]. Acad Emerg Med 2001;8:429.

26. Tokish JM, Powell ET, Schlegel TF, et al. Ketorolac use in the National Football League - prevalence, efficacy, and adverse effects. Phys Sportsmed 2002;30:19–24.

27. Burd T, Hughes M, Anglen J. Heterotopic ossification prophylaxis increases the risk of long-bone non-union. J Bone Joint Surg 2003;85-B:700–5.

28. Chuchmach M, Brian R. Ex-USC player: painkiller injections caused heart attack. ABC News. ABC News Network 2013. Available at: http://abcnews.go.com/Blotter/risks-college-football-powerful-painkiller/story?id=18114915. Accessed August 3, 2015.

29. Easterbrook, Gregg. Painkillers, NFL's other big problem. 2014. Available at: http://espn.go.com/nfl/story/_/id/10975522/excerpt-painkillers-abuse-nfl-king-sports-gregg-easterbrook. August 1, 2015.

30. Matava MJ, Brater C, Gritter N, et al. Recommendations of the National Football League Physician Society task force on the use of Toradol ketorolac in the National Football League. Sports Health 2012;4:377–83.

31. Controlled substance schedules. Resources. U.S. Department of Justice. Available at: http://www.deadiversion.usdoj.gov/schedules/index.html#define. Accessed August 2, 2015.

32. Mosby's medical dictionary. 8th edition. Elsevier; 2009.

33. Kieffer BL, Evans CJ. Opioid receptors: from binding sites to visible molecules in vivo. Neuropharmacology 2009;56(Suppl 1):205–12.

34. Al-Hasani R, Bruchas MR. Molecular mechanisms of opioid receptor-dependent signaling and behavior. Anesthesiology 2011;115:1363–81.

35. Volkow ND. America's addiction to opioids: heroin and prescription drug abuse. Rockville (MD): National Institute on Drug Abuse; 2014. Available at: http://www.drugabuse.gov/about-nida/legislative-activities/testimony-to-congress/2015/americas-addiction-to-opioids-heroin-prescription-drug-abuse. Accessed August 2, 2015.

36. Benyamin R, Trescot A, Datta S, et al. Opioid consumption and side effects. Pain Physician 2008;11(2 Supplement):S105–20.

37. DEA/Drug Scheduling. U.S. Drug Enforcement Agency. Available at: http://www.dea.gov/druginfo/ds.shtml. Accessed August 02, 2015.

38. Katz WA. Pharmacology and clinical experience with tramadol in osteoarthritis. Drugs 1996;52(Suppl 3):39–47.

39. Rules - 2014. Placement of tramadol into schedule IV. U.S. Department of Justice; 2014. Available at: http://www.deadiversion.usdoj.gov/fed_regs/rules/2014/fr0702.htm. Accessed August 03, 2015.

40. National Center for Health Statistics. United States, 2006 with chart book on trends in the health of Americans. Hyattsville (MD): NCHS; 2006. p. 68–71.

41. International Narcotics Control Board Report 2008. United Nations Pubns; 2009. p. 20.

42. Substance Abuse and Mental Health Services Administration. Results from the 2012 national survey on drug use and health: summary of national findings. NSDUH Series H-46, HHS Publication No. (SMA) 13–4795. Rockville (MD): Substance Abuse and Mental Health Services Administration; 2013.

43. Cotler L, Abdallah B, Cummings S, et al. Injury, pain, and prescription opioid use among former National Football League (NFL) players. Drug Alcohol Depend 2011;116:188–94.

44. American Council on Science and Health. Athletes being given narcotics so they can play through injuries? Dangerous, unethical, perhaps criminal? New York: American Council on Science and Health; 2015. Available at: http://acsh.org/2015/03/athletes-given-narcotics-can-play-injuries-dangerous-unethical-perhaps-criminal. Accessed August 2, 2015.

45. Darrow CJ, Collins CL, Yard EE, et al. Epidemiology of severe injuries among United States high school athletes: 2005–2007. Am J Sports Med 2009;37: 1798–805.

46. Veliz PT, Boyd C, McCabe SE. Playing through pain: sports participation and nonmedical use of opioid medications among adolescents. Am J Public Health 2013;103:e28–30.

47. Nepple JJ, Matava MJ. Soft tissue injections in the athlete. Sports Health 2009;1: 396–404.

48. Smith BJ, Collina SJ. Pain medications in the locker room - to dispense or not. Curr Sports Med Rep 2007;6:367–70.

49. Orchard JW. Benefits and risks of using local anaesthetic for pain relief to allow early return to play in professional football. Br J Sports Med 2002;36:209–13.

50. Parsons J. 2014-15 NCAA sports medicine handbook. Muhlenberg.edu. Indianapolis (IN): NCAA; 2014. Available at: http://www.muhlenberg.edu/pdf/main/athletics/athletic_training/2014_15_Sports_Medicine_Handbook.pdf. Accessed August 02, 2015.

51. Orchard J. Is it safe to use local anesthetic painkilling injections in professional football. Sports Med 2004;34:209–19.

Team Physicians, Sports Medicine, and the Law

An Update

Dionne L. Koller, JD, MA

KEYWORDS

• Sports medicine • Team physicians • Medical malpractice • Tort law • Athletes

KEY POINTS

- The practice of sports medicine and the work of team physicians are more important now than ever before.
- Millions of children and adults engage in sports, and state and federal legislatures are taking on sports medicine issues and seeking to regulate sports safety.
- The recognition of sports medicine and promulgation of practice guidelines for team physicians will push general medical malpractice standards to evolve into a more specialized standard of care for those who practice in this area.
- The sports medicine community should continue to think beyond the construct of tort law and malpractice liability.
- Sports medicine providers should look for opportunities to use medical knowledge and expertise to work within sports organizations to seek changes to the games when necessary to protect the health and well-being of athletes.

INTRODUCTION

The medicolegal issue that many physicians and attorneys think about often is malpractice liability. In the sports medicine context, however, this issue is not always the most legally significant. Although the work of team physicians and the practice of sports medicine have expanded, there are few reported cases of malpractice liability. Moreover, tort law applied to sports medicine remains largely unchanged. The same negligence standards that apply to the practice of medicine are generally used to evaluate medical care provided to athletes within a sports setting. Thus, from the medical malpractice standpoint, acting as a team physician or sports medicine specialist has no greater legal significance today than it did more than a decade ago.

Notably, however, state legislatures have identified the practice of sports medicine and the work of team physicians as presenting important policy issues to be

Center for Sport and the Law, University of Baltimore School of Law, 1401 North Charles Street, Baltimore, MD, USA
E-mail address: dkoller@ubalt.edu

Clin Sports Med 35 (2016) 245–255
http://dx.doi.org/10.1016/j.csm.2015.10.005
0278-5919/16/$ – see front matter

addressed. As this article explains, team physicians and sports medicine providers would be well served by familiarizing themselves not just with the standard of care for their specialty, but also any duties or obligations that are created by statute.

THE LEGAL SIGNIFICANCE OF BEING A TEAM PHYSICIAN AND PRACTICING SPORTS MEDICINE

Sports medicine is a term that applies to all those who provide health care services to athletes. Thus, sports medicine providers include athletic trainers, physical therapists, chiropractors, and physicians of varying specialties. Within the sports medicine team, the team physician takes a leadership role. Team physicians are usually primary care or family practice physicians or orthopedic surgeons who are hired by professional teams, colleges, and universities to provide medical care for their athletes. Many high schools also designate a physician to provide medical care to their athletes.[1] Team physicians may be compensated for the care they provide to athletes or render such services free of charge, a distinction that many state statutes make for purposes of granting malpractice immunity.

In general, the practice of sports medicine is not specially recognized in the context of tort law, and team physicians do not carry any special legal duties. However, given the regulation of sports, especially at the youth, interscholastic, and intercollegiate levels, there are potential areas of liability specifically concerning team physicians. Thus, team physicians must comply with applicable federal, state, and local law and regulations, as would any physician, and team physicians also must comply with any applicable school, league, or governing body guidelines.

Malpractice Liability

Given the variety of physicians who practice sports medicine and serve as team physicians, it is important that each understand his or her duties and the relevant standard of care for his or her specialty. In general, to establish a claim for medical negligence, an athlete must show that the physician had a duty of care as a result of a physician–patient relationship. The athlete must also establish that the physician breached that duty and that the physician's breach of his or her duty caused the athlete actual harm or damage.

A legal duty is established when the athlete can show that a physician–patient relationship exists. Such a relationship may exist for the team physician in the context of preparticipation physical examinations as well as for the diagnosis and treatment of injuries and for providing an athlete with medical clearance to return to play.[1] In general, the team physician's responsibility is to protect athletes' health and safety. The team physician, therefore, must provide medical care and advice that is in the athlete's best health interests.[1] The team physician must do this while navigating what may be difficult pressures from coaches, team administrators, parents, fans, and the athlete. Thus, when treating athletes, team physicians must keep in mind federal privacy laws such as the Health Insurance Portability and Accountability Act (HIPPA) and, for those treating student athletes, the Family Educational Rights and Privacy Act (FERPA), and not share an athlete's health information unless it is legally permissible. Moreover, although the team physician must not unnecessarily restrict an athlete's ability to play, the team physician must not allow his or her medical judgment to be affected by the team's need for the athlete to return or the athlete's desire to play.[2] Indeed, within the legal literature, the most frequently discussed issue involving team physicians and the practice of sports medicine is the potential for a conflict of interest that can corrupt a team physician's medical judgment and put an athlete's health at risk.[2,3]

To determine whether the physician breached his or her duty to an athlete–patient, courts will look to the relevant standard of care. The standard of care generally is that a physician must exercise the degree of care ordinarily possessed by members of the medical profession.[4] In addition, a team physician has a duty to disclose material information relevant to the athlete's play and in light of the athlete's physical condition. Thus, courts have held team physicians liable for failing to disclose material risks of play.[5]

The law looks to the medical profession to establish the standard of care by which a particular physician's treatment will be judged under the circumstances.[4] Therefore, evidence of the standard of care will come from practice guidelines, medical literature, and what is customary practice for a physician under similar circumstances. In a specific case, the plaintiff has the burden of producing expert testimony that articulates the applicable standard of care and that the physician breached the standard of care. For example, in *Zimbauer v Milwaukee Orthopedic Group, LTD.*, the court dismissed a professional baseball player's claim against his treating physician for allegedly misdiagnosing and treating a shoulder injury because the court held that the plaintiff failed to produce a physician expert who would testify to the appropriate standard of care and that the treating physician breached the standard of care.[6]

Because many different specialists act as team physicians—internists, pediatricians, and most often, orthopedic surgeons—the standard of care for team physicians is to conform to the standard of "good medical practice" by exercising the degree of skill and care that would be exhibited by a physician with similar specialty training.[1,7] Courts have not recognized sports medicine as a separate medical specialty with its own standard of care. As a result, liability is determined on a case-by-case basis, with applicable standards corresponding to the relevant physician's specialty.[1]

For instance, in *Gibson v Digiglia*, a professional hockey player brought suit against the team physician for damages resulting from the treatment of an eye injury.[8] The team physician was not present but was contacted by the player's coach and informed of the injury. The team physician spoke with the physicians who were providing care to the athlete, and those physicians cleared the athlete to be discharged from the hospital, fly home, and seek additional treatment. The athlete alleged that the delay in treatment of his eye injury coupled with the change in air pressure on the flight home caused him significant injury.

The court entered judgment for the team physician before the case went to the jury. The court rejected the plaintiff's argument that the team physician fell below the appropriate standard of care in authorizing the athlete's discharge and transfer home for additional care. The team physician argued that he relied on the assurances of the physicians who were treating the athlete in authorizing the transfer home. Importantly, although the plaintiff argued that the team physician had a duty to obtain the athlete's test results and medical records and confirm the accuracy of the opinions given by the treating physicians, the court rejected this argument. The court stated that the plaintiff presented no evidence to establish a "team physician" standard of care or that the team physician fell below the standard of care by relying on the information provided by the treating physicians.[10] The court found that the plaintiffs had presented no evidence that the team physician had a duty to confirm the accuracy of the information provided to him by the athlete's treating physician.

Other physicians have used specialists with sports medicine expertise to defend a malpractice allegation and defeat an athlete's claim. For example, in *Hamilton v Winder*, a professional hockey player alleged that the team physician negligently diagnosed and treated his elbow injury.[9] The court allowed the physician to use an "expert in sports medicine" to establish the standard of care for treating a suspected elbow infection. Similarly, in *Villegas v Feder*, an athlete brought suit against a team physician for clearing him to play collegiate football and treating his ankle injury.[10] The team physician was a board-certified family physician who had completed a sports medicine fellowship. To support his defense that he adhered to the standard of care, the team physician produced the opinion of a board-certified internist who held a Certificate of Added Qualification in sports medicine and who was a team physician certified by the American College of Sports Medicine. The defendant's expert testified that the team physician properly relied on the athlete's representation that the athlete's orthopedic surgeon had cleared the athlete to play football. The athlete–plaintiff submitted the testimony of a board-certified orthopedic surgeon. The court held that although the orthopedic surgeon was qualified to render an opinion on the care of the athlete's ankle, the orthopedic surgeon could not give an opinion on whether the athlete should have been cleared to play football. The court stated that the athlete's expert did not state that he had "any specific training or expertise in evaluating a student's fitness to participate in collegiate athletics for an educational institution" and did not indicate that the expert had "familiarized himself with the relevant literature, standards of care or protocol applicable to that procedure."[13] The team physician was, therefore, able to defeat the athlete's claim.

Malpractice litigation in this area is also affected by state statutes. Some states have statutes that address the issue of the appropriate expert opinion testimony that may be used in a medical malpractice action. These statutes may permit a wider range of expert testimony against those acting as team physicians. For instance, in *Weiss v Pratt*, a high school football player brought a medical malpractice claim against an orthopedic surgeon who served as a volunteer team physician for a high school football team.[11] The team physician appealed the judgment against him on the grounds that the trial court erred in allowing an emergency room physician to render expert testimony regarding the team physician's treatment of the athlete while the athlete was still on the football field, because the emergency physician was neither an orthopedic surgeon nor a team physician. The defendant team physician argued that the state's immunity statute for volunteer team physicians and the state's medical malpractice expert testimony statute required an expert witness in the same specialty as the physician against whom the testimony was being offered.[12] Moreover, the team physician argued that the statute governing expert witness testimony in medical malpractice actions required testimony from a physician in a "similar specialty." The court held that the team physician immunity statute required only a "similarly licensed" physician to testify as an expert. The court stated that "even though the expert witness has never served as a volunteer team physician, never treated an athlete on the field, never practiced orthopedic surgery, and was not board certified, he was 'similarly licensed'" because both the defendant team physician and the expert were medical doctors.

The court also held that the medical malpractice expert witness testimony statute did not require the expert to be in the exact same specialty as the team physician defendant. Although the court stated that its decision was based on "the specific facts" of the case, it held that testimony from an emergency physician about the team physician's care of the athlete on the field was appropriate. Specifically, the court stated that even though the emergency physician was not an orthopedic surgeon, because the emergency physician "had the expertise of what to do" on the football field, where the athlete had suffered a possible spinal cord injury and was not placed on a backboard, the court held the testimony was admissible. The court did state, however, that if the athlete's allegations of malpractice had concerned an aspect of orthopedic surgery requiring "a specific level of specialization," the emergency physician may not have been qualified to render an opinion.

Also of note from the *Weiss* case is that the court raised questions for the legislature about the team physician immunity statute. The statute provided, in pertinent part, that any individual licensed to practice medicine who is acting in the capacity of a volunteer team physician who agrees to gratuitously provide care at an athletic event sponsored by an elementary or secondary school may not be held liable for such treatment. The statute specified that the immunity applied where the care provided "was rendered as a reasonably prudent person similarly licensed to practice medicine would have acted under the same or similar circumstances."[13] The court in *Weiss* remarked that the statute, "while purporting to immunize a volunteer physician," provided "little more protection than general tort law," and that the statute's protection was "illusory." The Florida legislature responded by amending the statute to provide that there will be no liability unless the treatment provided "was rendered in a wrongful manner." The statute further defines "wrongful manner" as being "in bad faith or with malicious purpose or in a manner exhibiting wanton and willful disregard of human rights, safety or property." This revised standard does provide significantly more protection for team physicians than general tort law. However, team physicians should be mindful that other state statutes seeking to immunize volunteer team physicians may not be drafted in a way that provides additional protection beyond the requirements of general tort law.

Given the use of team physicians at nearly all levels of sport and the development of standards for those who act as team physicians, future litigation likely will see an evolution in the standard of care to more specifically account for the special training and focus of physicians practicing in the sports context, rather than simply having the standard of care remain tethered only to the physician's specialty area.

Statutes

Although there has been little case law that directly addresses the duties of team physicians, state legislatures have been active in proposing or enacting measures that address issues arising in this context. Legislatures have enacted statutes addressing three areas: team physician immunity, team physician travel, and specific requirements for sports medicine care. Moreover, nearly all states regulate athletic trainers.

Immunity

State immunity statutes for team physicians are aimed primarily at youth and amateur sports. These statutes seek to provide malpractice immunity for physicians acting as volunteers in connection with school or other amateur sports organized for children. Although the provisions all seek to protect team physicians from liability, they are varied in scope. Some states, such as Florida (described above) and Ohio, provide immunity for a volunteer team physician unless he or she engaged in willful or wanton misconduct.[14] States such as Louisiana provide immunity unless the athlete can show that the injury was the result of "gross negligence."[15] Other states, such as California, limit immunity to certain categories of athletic events.[16] Some states are more expansive, providing immunity for team "volunteer health providers" as part of more comprehensive immunity provisions that apply to volunteer athletic coaches and officials. States such as Georgia expand the immunity to include preseason physical examinations, and liability will accrue only where the physician engaged in a "willful or wanton act" or if the physician failed to take action to provide or arrange for further medical treatment.[17]

Other types of statutory immunity include provisions for physicians who supervise or direct athletic trainers. For example, Arizona enacted a statute requiring that athletic trainers be directed in general practice by a team physician or other licensed physician, and that such physician who, without compensation, provides "recommendations, guidelines and instructions as to standard protocols to be followed in the general day-to-day activities in which athletic trainers engage" is not subject to liability unless the physician acted with gross negligence or engaged in intentional misconduct.[18]

Team physician travel

Another area in which legislatures are enacting law to account for sports medicine is in the area of team physician travel. Because sports at nearly all levels are no longer "local" or limited to in-state competition, states have recognized the need for teams to travel with their physicians. As a result, many states have proposed or enacted legislation that provides protections for visiting team physicians. Such legislation provides a waiver of state medical licensing requirements while the physician is present in a state in which he or she is not licensed to practice medicine for purposes of providing medical services to a team that is participating in an athletic event in the state. Thus, several states have statutes exempting physicians from applicable licensing requirements if they have an agreement to provide medical care to a sports team and the team is traveling to the state for an event.[19] These statutes generally require that the team physician have an agreement with a sports team or otherwise be officially designated by the team as its team physician; that the team physician limit his or her care to the team's athletes, officials, and coaching staff; and that the physician will not enjoy practice privileges in any of the state's health care facilities.

There is also a bill currently pending in Congress that if enacted would address this issue. The proposed Sports Medicine Licensure Clarity Act would deem that a team physician's services, when provided in a state in which the team physician is not licensed to practice medicine, are provided in the state in which the team physician is licensed to practice medicine. The proposed statute's provisions would apply for purposes of determining the team physician's liability insurance coverage and civil and criminal malpractice liability in circumstances in which the team physician is traveling to provide medical services to a sports team.[20]

Required care/injury management

Perhaps the most significant legislative effort in the area of sports medicine in recent years is the enactment of state statutes requiring proper management of youth athletes who are suspected of sustaining a concussion. Between 2009 and 2014, every state and the District of Columbia enacted legislation that focused on mitigating the harm of concussions and returning to play too soon.[21] All of these measures require an athlete to be removed from play if a concussion is suspected and require appropriate medical clearance before an athlete returns to play. State statutes vary widely, however, in designating which medical providers are competent to certify that an athlete is fit to return to play. Most statutes specify that only a "licensed health care provider trained in the evaluation and management of concussion" may clear an athlete to return to play.[22] Others simply provide that a "licensed health care professional" may clear an athlete to return to play.[23] The types of health care professionals listed as being competent to clear an athlete to return to play range from licensed physicians to nurse practitioners, physician assistants, athletic trainers, and neuropsychologists. Additionally, some statutes provide at least qualified immunity for physicians or others who clear an athlete to return to play.[24] However, other statutes may create liability in situations in which a physician clears an athlete to return to play but the physician did not have adequate training to make such an assessment.[25]

Like the movement to address concussions in sports, states are also showing an interest in legislating standards for preparticipation physicals, specifically to require screening for cardiac conditions. For example, New Jersey requires a preparticipation cardiac screening and also requires that a health care provider (including physicians and physician assistants) who performs preparticipation physical examinations must complete a "Student-Athlete Cardiac Screening professional development module."[26] Other states, such as Illinois, have considered proposals to include a screening of all individuals younger than 19 years for cardiac conditions as outlined in the Preparticipation Physical Evaluation Form.[27]

EMERGING LEGAL ISSUES

Among the many issues that are important to team physicians and the sports medicine community, 2 stand out as being the most legally significant at this time. The concussion issue at all levels and across a range of sports remains an issue on state and federal policy agendas, and the legal implications of this issue are not yet fully known. In addition, the issue of prescription drug use, especially in the context of professional sports, became very prominent in the last year, and it remains to be seen what further legal issues will develop.

Concussions

Over the last several years, the sports medicine legal issue that has dominated the headlines has been concussions—both preventing and managing them—at all levels and across a range of sports. The issue of sports-related concussions will remain legally significant beyond the recent flurry of litigation and legislative activity. In terms of liability, the bulk of litigation brought over concussions has been against sports teams, leagues, and sponsoring institutions. High profile cases against the National Football League and the National Collegiate Athletic Association have settled, and numerous other suits against groups such as Pop Warner, US Soccer, and high school athletic associations have been dismissed or are likely to be dismissed because of issues of causation and immunity.

However, although sports leagues and other sponsoring entities may not be as easily liable for harm to athletes from sports concussions, physicians practicing in the sports context still do face legal liability for failing to properly manage an athlete's concussion. State statutes and relevant athletic program guidelines put greater emphasis than ever before on physicians detecting and properly managing athlete's concussions. As such, physicians must be aware of current medical practices in this area. Guidelines such as the *Consensus Statement on Concussion in Sport*,[28] the Centers for Disease Control's Heads Up "toolkit" for physicians, and those published by groups such as the American Academy of Neurology and the American Academy of Pediatrics will all be relevant in determining the standard of care in litigation involving athletes who have suffered a concussion. Significantly, current concussion management guidelines are aimed not just at specialists such as neurologists, but all health care providers who may come in contact with an athlete suffering from a concussion. As such, it will be difficult for team physicians to make the argument in malpractice litigation involving an athlete with a concussion that such knowledge was outside the scope of the physician's specialty.

What remains to be determined as a matter of tort liability is whether a physician has a duty to remove an athlete from a game, or not allow an athlete to return to play, when the athlete is suspected of having a concussion but does not complain of symptoms and seeks to return to play. Team physicians are aware of the pressures on athletes to remain in the game, especially at the collegiate and professional levels. However, courts have generally not been willing to hold coaches and others accountable for an athlete's injuries when an athlete has not made clear that he or she is hurt. For instance, in *Zemke v Arreola*, a high school football player sued his coach and the school system for allowing him to return to play after suffering a head injury. The court noted that the athlete did not complain of a headache or other injury related to his head but only stated that he had suffered a finger injury. The team physician on the sidelines of the game cleared the athlete to return to play, and the athlete subsequently suffered a subdural hematoma. The court found it pivotal that the athlete had not reported symptoms consistent with a head injury to the team physician or athletic trainer.[29] In contrast, in *Scottland v Duva Boxing LLC*, the court held that the ringside physician had a duty to exercise reasonable medical judgment and terminate the match if necessary to protect a boxer's well-being.[30] Although this holding was based on the standard set by statutes regulating boxing, team physicians should be mindful of statutes and medical guidelines that could prescribe taking action when a concussion is suspected, regardless of whether an athlete reports symptoms.

Finally, because state youth concussion statutes vary widely in designating which medical providers are competent to certify that an athlete is fit to return to play, physicians practicing in this area should expect additional legislative clarification over which types of providers may, and may not, certify that an athlete to return to play. Moreover, physicians should be aware that researchers have found significant issues with parents "doctor shopping" or seeking opinions from numerous physicians to find one who will clear the child–athlete for play.[6]

Prescription of Drugs

With respect to prescription drugs, 2 legal issues are currently of concern for team physicians. The first is improperly prescribing or dispensing prescription drugs to keep athletes in the game and available to play. The second is team physicians traveling with prescription drugs, including controlled substances.

In general, team physicians have a duty to inform an athlete of the risks of playing in light of the athlete's condition, and the team physician should only prescribe medication to enable continued play if doing so is consistent with the athlete's health interests.[1] Team physicians can be held liable for negligently prescribing cortisone, pain killers, and other medications to facilitate an athlete's participation in sports while injured.[5]

In addition, when prescribing medication to athletes, team physicians must comply with all relevant laws regarding possessing and dispensing drugs.[1] These include the Controlled Substances Act, 21 U.S.C. §§ 801 *et seq*. and the accompanying federal regulations, the Federal Food, Drug, and Cosmetic Act, 21 U.S.C. §331(d), and state laws on prescription drugs. For instance, the Controlled Substances Act and state law contain several provisions regarding the dispensation, possession, and use of prescription drugs. Team physicians who travel outside of their state of licensure must be careful to ensure that they are properly handling and dispensing medication. Moreover, team physicians should not delegate to athletic trainers the authority to dispense controlled substances.

These issues became prominent in the last year. In 2014, a group of former National Football League (NFL) players brought suit against the league in the case of *Dent v National Football League*. The plaintiffs alleged that, among other things, team physicians, athletic trainers, and other staff violated applicable prescription drug laws by dispensing drugs, including controlled substances, without proper prescriptions, failing to keep appropriate records, and using athletic trainers to dispense controlled substances. The case was dismissed because the court held that the claims were preempted by the NFL's collective bargaining agreement. The case is on appeal, and a decision is expected by the end of the year. Several months after the lawsuit was filed, the federal Drug Enforcement Administration conducted a surprise raid on several NFL team medical staffs as part of its investigation into prescription drug abuse in the league. The Drug Enforcement Administration reportedly had concerns that NFL teams were dispensing drugs in violation of the Controlled Substances Act to keep players in the game.

Although to some extent these issues are arguably being addressed at the state level, with legislation authorizing team physicians to practice medicine outside of the state of licensure, those measures do not address potential issues that might arise under federal law. To date, Congress has not taken action that would clarify these issues for team physicians or others who travel out of state with controlled substances and other prescription medication and the legal implications of traveling with such medication remains unclear.

SUMMARY

The practice of sports medicine and the work of team physicians are more important now than ever before. Millions of children and adults engage in sports, and state and federal legislatures are taking on sports medicine issues and seeking to regulate sports safety. Moreover, the recognition of sports medicine and promulgation of practice guidelines for team physicians will push general medical malpractice standards to evolve into a more specialized standard of care for those who practice in this area. As a result, those involved in the sports medicine community would be served by 2 strategies. First, sports medicine providers should continue to engage in meaningful efforts to educate lawmakers, especially at the state level, on the role of team physicians and the important issues that impact the practice of medicine in the sports context. Importantly, sports medicine professionals can help policymakers understand which issues are appropriate for legislative action and which are not. Second, the sports medicine community should continue working to define the practice of sports medicine and duties and obligations of team physicians. To the extent that practicing medicine in the sports context involves calculations that do not arise in typical medical practice, the sports medicine community can help elucidate those issues and create appropriate guidelines that can serve to inform athlete–patients and educate courts. Doing so will help best set the terms by which those who practice sports medicine are judged.

Finally, the sports medicine community should continue to think beyond the construct of tort law and malpractice liability. Sports medicine providers should look for opportunities to use medical knowledge and expertise to work within sports organizations to seek changes to the games when necessary to protect the health and well-being of athletes. Rather than take sports as currently constructed as a given, sports medicine providers can provide much needed leadership and be an important force for positive evolution of the sports we know and love.

REFERENCES

1. Mitten MJ. Emerging legal issues in sports medicine: a synthesis, summary, and analysis, vol. 76. St. John's L. Rev. 2002. p. 5.
2. Calandrillo SP. Sports medicine conflicts: team physicians vs. athlete-patients, vol. 50. St. Louis U.L.J.; 2005. p. 185.
3. Furrow BR. Health law symposium: the problem of the sports doctor: serving two (or is it three or four?) masters, vol. 50. St. Louis U.L.J.; 2005. p. 165.

4. Mitten MJ. Annotation, medical malpractice liability of sports medicine care providers for injury to, or death of, athletes, vol. 33. 5th edition. ALR: p. 619.
5. Krueger v. San Francisco Forty Niners, 234 Cal. Rptr. 579 (Cal. Ct. App. 1987).
6. Zimbauer v. Milwaukee Orthopedic Group, LTD vol. 920 F.Suppl 959, 967 E.D.Wis. 1996).
7. Landis M. The team physician: an analysis of the causes of action, conflicts, defenses and improvements, vol. 1. In: Depaul J, editor. Sports L Contemp Probs. 2003. p. 139.
8. Gibson v. Digiglia, 980 So. 2d 739, 741 (La.App. 3 Cir. 2008).
9. Hamilton v. Winder, 2007 La. App. Unpub. LEXIS 432 (La. App. 1 Cir. 5/4/07).
10. Villegas v. Feder, 901 N.Y.S.2d 911 (2009).
11. Weiss v. Pratt, 53 So.3d 395 (Fla.App. 4 Dist. 2011).
12. The statutes at issue in Weiss were Fla. Sta. §768.135 (volunteer team physicians immunity) and Fla. Stat. §766.102 (expert witness testimony in medical malpractice actions).
13. Fla. Stat. §768.135.
14. ORC Ann. 2305.231(B); M.S.A. §604A.11 (immunity unless acts were committed in a "willful and wanton or reckless manner.").
15. LSA-R.S. 9:2798.
16. Cal. Ed. Code §49409 (interscholastic athletic events); Va. Code Ann. §8.01–225.1; W.Va. Code §55-7-19(b). Similarly, Oregon provides protections for team physicians rendering emergency care not just at interscholastic athletic events, but also college and "other athletic events." ORS §30.800(b)(2).
17. O.C.G.A. §51-1-45.
18. A.R.S. §;32–4103.
19. Cal. Bus. & Prof. Code §2076; S.C. Code Ann. §40-47-30(B)(1)(c); Va. Code Ann. §54.1-2901(A)(30).
20. S.689, 114th Cong. (2015-2016).
21. Harvey HH, Koller DL, Lowrey KM. The four stages of youth sports TBI policymaking: engagement, enactment, research, and reform. J Law Med Ethics 2015; 43(1):87.
22. West's Revised Code of Wash. Ann. 28A.600.190(4); North Dakota Century Code Annotated §15.1–18.2-04(4).
23. Neb. Rev. St. §71–9104(2)(a); 16 V.S.A. §1431(d)(2)(requiring written permission from a "health care provider."); South Carolina Code 1976 §59-63-75(d)(3)(requiring medical clearance by a "physician.").
24. West's Revised Code of Wash. Ann. 28A.600.190(4). (providing for liability only if the volunteer health care provider engaged in willful or wanton misconduct or acts that constitute gross negligence); Tenn. Code Ann. §68-55-503(b)(3)(no liability when health care provider is acting "in good faith"; does not cover acts of "willful misconduct," "gross negligence," or "reckless disregard."); South Carolina Code 1976 §59-63-75(d)(5)(extending immunity to athletic trainers, physicians, physician assistants or nurse practitioners who serve as volunteers and do not engage in gross negligence or willful or wanton misconduct).
25. North Dakota Century Code Annotated §15.1-18.2-04(5)(c)(stating that "any health care provider who signs an authorization… is acknowledging that the provider is acting within the provider's scope of practice and is trained in the evaluation and management of concussion, as determined by the provider's licensing board).
26. N.J.S.A. 18A:40-41.7; N.J.S.A. 26:2–192(a)(effective Sept. 1, 2015).
27. 2015 Ill. Senate Bill No. 8, Ill. 99th Gen. Assembly (January 15, 2015).

28. McCrory P, Meeuwisse WH, Aubry M, et al. Consensus statement on concussion in sport: the 4th international conference on concussion in sport held in Zurich, November 2012, Br J Sports Med 2013;47:250–8.
29. Zemke v. Arreola, 2006 Cal. App. Unpub. LEXIS 4999.
30. Scottland v. Duva Boxing LLC, 2005 N.Y.Misc. LEXIS 8482 (2005).

Concussion Ethics and Sports Medicine

Michael J. McNamee, BA, MA, MA, PhD[a],*, Bradley Partridge, BSc, PhD[b], Lynley Anderson, MSc, PhD[c]

KEYWORDS

- Concussion • Mild traumatic brain injury • Conflicts of interest • Rugby union
- Australian football • Rugby league

KEY POINTS

- Compared with many other branches of sports medicine, concussion diagnosis and management science and clinical practice are in their early stages of development.
- The complexity of the neurologic conditions and the lack of consensus over them compound this observation.
- Although leading concussion experts have identified what they take to be best practice, numerous problems remain in its implementation across the sports spectrum.

INTRODUCTION

Over the past 15 years there has been a proliferation of position statements and professional guidelines published on sports concussion management.[1–4] Some of these statements have had considerable influence over professional sporting leagues and governing bodies—for example, the Australian Football League, National Rugby League (NRL), and World Rugby (formerly the International Rugby Board) have all modeled their concussion policies on the most recent consensus statements[5,6] published by the self-appointed group of experts known as the Concussion in Sport Group. Accordingly, various leagues have mandated the use of tools recommended by consensus statements to aid assessors in the recognition of concussion (eg, the Sport Concussion Assessment Tool—3rd Edition [SCAT3]) and to monitor recovery (eg, computerized neuropsychological tests), and over time there has also been a move toward a no same-day return-to-play (RTP) policy for athletes diagnosed with concussion, which has gained widespread acceptance across sports.

The consensus statements make it clear that decision making about concussion is still ultimately within the realm of clinical judgment and that "management and return

[a] College of Engineering, Swansea University, Singleton Park, Swansea SA1 8QQ, UK; [b] Faculty of Health and Behavioural Sciences, The University of Queensland, St Lucia, Queensland QLD 4072, Australia; [c] Division of Health Sciences, University of Otago, Dunedin 9016, New Zealand
* Corresponding author.
E-mail address: m.j.mcnamee@swansea.ac.uk

Clin Sports Med 35 (2016) 257–267
http://dx.doi.org/10.1016/j.csm.2015.10.008
0278-5919/16/$ – see front matter © 2016 Elsevier Inc. All rights reserved.

to play (RTP) decisions remain in the realm of clinical judgment on an individualised basis."[6] It is acceptable in principle then that the recommendations of concussion guidelines may ultimately be overruled by clinical judgment. But amid the increased adoption of formal procedures that assessors must follow when dealing with potentially concussed athletes (which in many US States has culminated in legislation), clinicians are confronted with considerable conceptual, empirical, and ethical uncertainty when diagnosing and managing concussion.[7]

Despite a long list of potential symptoms and signs of concussion and the existence of various recognition tools that have been developed, there is no consensus on when a concussion diagnosis must apply. In philosophic terms, there are no logically necessary and sufficient conditions for the concept of *concussion* – not even the obvious candidate: loss of consciousness. The lack of consensus over definition is likely to compound the validity and reliability of prevalence data – which are of fundamental importance as scientists, clinicians, and athletes (not to mention franchises and health insurers) attempting to gain a firmer grasp on the nature and scope of the problem.

Notwithstanding the implementation of formal concussion management policies and protocols by many sports governing bodies, there is almost no guidance on how clinicians should navigate ethical issues that arise. Some of the most difficult issues confronting team doctors and sporting leagues regarding head trauma are those arising from the competing interests of stakeholders.[8–10] Part of this uncertainty arises from a reasonable concern regarding how concussion guidelines should be interpreted in the light of the demands and potential risks of different sports. These problems are compounded when the decisions made by physicians are not supported by the relevant organization to whom they offer their services – whether voluntarily or professionally.

The authors' concern is with a set of interconnected ethical issues. First, problems are discussed arising from identification, diagnosis, and management guidelines. Secondly, issues of conflicts of interest within the profession of sports medicine and how these may bring about coercive or undue influence in the decisions regarding diagnosis and RTP are considered. Third, the specific problem of same-day RTP for head-injured athletes is discussed. Fourth, ethical issues concerned with reporting and auditing head injuries and what rights athletes might be expected to enjoy in relation to their injury history qua concussion are discussed. Fifth, the extent to which independent match day doctors (MDDs) might address some concerns about conflicts of interest in the context of professional sports is discussed. The authors conclude that position statements notwithstanding, there is much that sports governing bodies should do to better guide their members – and sports communities more generally – in relation to the various processes attending concussion, from injury to (safe) RTP.

PROBLEMS IN THE IDENTIFICATION AND DIAGNOSIS OF CONCUSSION, UNCERTAINTY ABOUT REPEATED CONCUSSIONS

Given that the term, *head injury*, covers a multitude of events, the medico-scientific community would be expected to have acted on the need for greater specification. The term with widest application is *mild traumatic brain injury (mTBI)* but this too covers a multitude of injuries and specifies only the level of injury. Concussion, although more specific, is still contested as a concept in medical science and practice. Vagnozzi and colleagues[11] claim, "there are still no standard criteria for the diagnosis and treatment for this peculiar condition." They identify 2 different approaches to mTBI focusing on direct mechanical trauma and subsequent biochemical sequelae.

The methods of identification and diagnosis of these phenomena are distinct and it may be difficult to reconcile them. Direct trauma and its mechanical effects may be apparent on or about the time of injury, whereas subsequent changes in brain chemistry may take longer to be identified.

A further complication arises when subsequent head injuries occur while an athlete patient may be considered especially vulnerable after a concussion. Vagnozzi and colleagues[11] argue that it is repeated insults to the brain that are potentially more troubling although medico-scientific consensus is not settled regarding the amount of time the brain of an athlete might be compromised by a first blow; thus, the time window of vulnerability to more sustained harm by further insults to the brain is especially important to determine. Some scientists have indicated a window of vulnerability that merits a 30-day recovery period,[12,13] but this view is not universally shared in the medico-scientific communities. Given individual differences in the nature of injury and its consequences, it is not clear how reliable this period is. The sporting consequences of such a layoff to professional athletes and teams, however, would be significant.

In addition, there are concerns about the long-term neurologic effects of repeated head trauma, given postmortem evidence of chronic traumatic encephalopathy (CTE) in dozens of former American football players.[14] Nevertheless, there has been considerable debate about the definition and etiology of CTE. For instance, the Consensus Statement on Concussion in Sport from the 4th International Conference on Concussion in Sport argues, "a cause and effect relationship has not as yet been demonstrated between CTE and concussion or exposure to contact sports."[6] This response is unsatisfactory for at least 2 reasons. First, cause-and-effect relations are not identifiable for a range of medical conditions but this does not prevent clinicians from acting on them. Second, the loose formulation of the second clause – that there is no proved causality between concussion and exposure to contact sports – is itself problematic. What constitutes "exposure"? And why would anyone think that mere "exposure" to contact sports was problematic qua concussion. Athletes might play a lifetime of contact sports and not experience concussion. This does not entail that CTE does not arise from repeated insults to the brain that some players are exposed to by virtue of their positional requirements or team strategy.

Given the emerging status of concussion science, it is unsurprising that there is variability in knowledge and practices regarding concussion within and across the sporting community. Knowledge about diagnosis and management is more likely to be available the higher an athlete has risen within a sport due to the presence and availability of health professionals on the sidelines. In the various subelite-level sports, athletes have to rely more heavily on team management, match officials, team members, and coaches who may or may not be suitably informed and who are unlikely to be professionally obligated to act in athletes' best interests.

The variability in knowledge about concussion can be compounded by a more general difficulty in identifying and diagnosing a concussion. Many times a suspected concussion is not straightforward to identify.[15] First, although most concussions are the result of a direct trauma to the head, not all are. Whiplash-type injuries, where a heavy blow to the torso forces a player's head to suffer a corresponding sudden deceleration or change in direction, may also cause a concussion.[6]

During the course of a game, there is potential for a concussion to be missed or underreported. At lower levels of sport where no health professionals are present, coaches, parents, referees, and others may raise concerns about a suspected concussion; however, their knowledge on concussion assessment and management can be assumed, at best, to be cursory.[16] An examination of the following chain of events demonstrates the number of ways in which a concussion may be missed.

Suppose a player receives a blow to the head. The first question to be asked is, Has this been observed or not? If so, then the player may be followed-up; if not, then the concussion may be missed. Yet, because of the variability in knowledge of concussion, even if the incident is observed, there is no guarantee given the skill set of those overseeing the activity that it will be recognized as a potential concussion.

If an incident is not observed by any of the personnel in positions of relevant authority or with a duty of care, a player may still report the injury. To be able to do this, players need to know of the importance of concussions, recognize that they have had such an injury, and understand the significance of it. Even if players do know these facts, they may be fearful of being prevented from playing and may not report the injury.[17] The lack of willingness to self-report is likely compounded by athletes who are marginal in the squad, whose position is under threat, or whose contract may be near its end.

If a concussion has been missed up to this point, there is still a chance that an injury may come to light if someone detects a subsequent behavior change in an athlete. At higher levels of the sport, baseline tests and knowledge of players can inform a team doctor or physiotherapist if an athlete displays signs of change in behavior. At lower levels of the sport, such baseline testing is not carried out, so determining abnormalities is difficult. Evidence in the form of knowledge of player behavior is important but rests on physician/athlete familiarity.

A head-injured athlete who is fortunate enough to have a clinician in attendance may undergo a SCAT3 test to help diagnose concussion. As evidenced on the SCAT3 test, it is doctors who are tasked with assessment and diagnosis of concussion, but this is not to say that doctors are the only health professional group with training in diagnosis and management of concussion. Some physiotherapists may also have received training on the topic of concussion during their undergraduate years and, more specifically, on sports-related concussion during sports physiotherapy education in both undergraduate and postgraduate studies. In some instances, it may be that an experienced sports physiotherapist is better placed to determine a concussion than a doctor who is unfamiliar with this sort of injury.

Even where there is knowledge and education on concussion, however, it cannot be assured that all these people have the best interest of the athlete at heart or the confidence to advocate on behalf of the athlete and challenge others around them who may be demanding that an athlete return to the field of play despite the injury. These issues are discussed.

CONFLICTS OF INTEREST AND COERCION

Medical professionals are required to exercise their clinical judgment on behalf of their patients under some conception of a patient's best interests. It has been argued that the first ethical duty of a sports physician is to act in the best interests of the athlete patient.[18] Yet many sports physicians also find themselves feeling obligated to serve the interests of the team (eg, club or franchise) they work for. This can manifest itself in several organizational structures where the physician is accountable to, for example, a coach or manager to whom the physician reports and whose performance objectives may influence medical decisions on capacity to play. For example, a New Zealand survey of sports medicine physicians found that a majority felt a sense of responsibility to the coach and to the team management.[19] As a result, in many professional sports settings, the traditional patient-doctor relationship is better characterized not as a dyad but rather as a triad of patient-doctor-team.[20] This relationship can give rise to a conflict of interest if a team doctor's assessment and judgment of the patient in that situation may tend to be less reliable than otherwise is the case.

At times, a team's/coach's interests may conflict with the welfare of an injured player (particularly if a coach wants a player to continue while injured), and it is well known that some coaches and managers do not always have player welfare as their top priority.[8] Over a significant period of time, research has demonstrated that athletes themselves are so committed to the norms of sport performance and identity that they fail to report or underreport symptoms, including those of concussion.[21] Although the methodologies for such evaluation are contested for reasons, such as memory recall bias, the general phenomenon is accepted. This arises not merely in the elite or professional domains but also is reported at high school level.[22,23] According to a recent report of the Institute of Medicine of the National Academies of Sciences, Engineering, and Medicine, "the culture of sports negatively influences athletes' self-reporting of concussion symptoms and their adherence to return-to-play guidance."[24]

In the recent past it has not been uncommon for players of many contact sports (including rugby union, American football, rugby league, and Australian rules football) to continue playing after being concussed, particularly if their symptoms did not prevent them from executing their roles on the field. The Consensus Statement on Concussion in Sport from the 3rd International Conference on Concussion in Sport allowed for the prospect that some professional athletes (such as National Football League [NFL] players) could rapidly RTP on the same day,[5] although that possibility has been (properly) ruled out in the Consensus Statement on Concussion in Sport from the 4th International Conference on Concussion in Sport.[6] In these situations, deciding whether to apply a diagnosis of concussion was perhaps not seen as crucial as deciding whether the symptoms of concussion were severe enough to prevent continued play. Cautious team doctors may have often faced pressure from coaches to permit players diagnosed with concussion to continue despite their symptoms. There are good reasons to believe that some coaches attempt to exert such pressure – for example, until recently the concussion guidelines of the NRL foreshadowed such attempts by stating, "The assessor should not be swayed by the opinion of the player, coaching staff or anyone else suggesting premature return to play."

Exercising good clinical judgment can be further complicated because there are often coercive pressures on players to underreport symptoms of concussion. These pressures may come from many stakeholders, including teammates, coaches, parents, and fans, and are not confined to professional athletes. A recent study of collegiate athletes found that 25% had experienced pressure to play on after a head injury and those who experienced such pressure had less intention to notify someone of a suspected concussion.[25] Worryingly, it seems that players are in turn a major source of pressure on team doctors. Kroshus and colleagues[26] found that among clinicians working with National Collegiate Athletic Association institutions, approximately two-thirds experienced pressure from players to prematurely clear them to RTP from concussion, and more than half of the surveyed clinicians experienced similar pressure from coaches.

SAME-DAY RETURN-TO-PLAY

The implementation of formal concussion rules within sporting leagues can in some cases increase these tensions among stakeholders, especially when breaches of these rules are backed with the prospect of sanctions. The clearest examples are rules prohibiting a player diagnosed with concussion from returning to play on the same day as the injury. Since some governing bodies have implemented the no same-day RTP rule, a considerable amount of tension has shifted onto whether an actual diagnosis of concussion should be applied in the first place (not simply whether a concussed athlete's symptoms have subsided). This is because in many amateur and professional sporting leagues a concussion diagnosis now automatically rules out further play regardless of whether the clinician believes an athlete's symptoms have resolved.

There have been several observable consequences. First, some clinicians seem to have initially seen these rules as an unnecessary or unwelcome encroachment on their clinical judgment, particularly in regard to determining recovery and the risks of continued participation. For example, one NRL team doctor explained,[27] "I am going to be pulling players out of the game who I have been comfortable letting continue for many years, and possibly hurting our team's chances of winning games."

This view implies 2 things: (1) in the past, some team doctors have used the leeway that clinical judgment allows to return a concussed player to the field on the same day and (2) team doctors are aware that their decisions about concussion can substantially affect the fortunes of the team they work for. It is precisely because team doctors may feel a sense of obligation or responsibility to the both the team/coach and their patient that this unease is felt.

Teams may experience a strategic disadvantage by having a player excluded because of a concussion diagnosis. In some sports, but not all, a substitute player may be brought on. Even here, however, anecdotal evidence suggests that some coaches have brought pressures on players to feign nonhead injury for treatment so that third parties are not aware that the reason for exclusion is likely concussion, so that they may be returned to play, if needed, for the short-term good of the team. This situation compromises the physician attempting to serve the patient's best interests. In soccer, Fédération Internationale de Football Association (FIFA) rules do not currently permit this. Four scenarios are discussed that reveal the heterogeneity and complexity of the current landscape of diagnosis and RTP.

First, one way that some teams have attempted to circumvent the potential disadvantage that arises from a player removed from the field of play is by ensuring that some players with a potential concussion are not examined by the team doctors so that a concussion diagnosis cannot be made. For example, several NRL teams have been sanctioned for failing to remove a player from the field to undergo a thorough concussion assessment by the team doctor even though the player exhibited symptoms of concussion (see, for example, Crawley[28]). If players are not assessed, then they cannot diagnosed with concussion and thus cannot be excluded from the field of play. In several instances, this practice was facilitated by allowing athletic trainers to briefly assess (and clear) players for concussion while they were still on the field despite these trainers not being qualified to diagnose concussion.[8]

Second, even in cases where qualified medical personnel have been allowed to assess players, questions remain about the influence of team goals on the assessor's decision. One well-known example in the United Kingdom's Premier League is Tottenham Hotspur Football Club goalkeeper Hugo Lloris, who was permitted to continue after exhibiting symptoms of concussion when team manager André Villas-Boas overruled medical staff.[29] A third, and more egregious, example occurred in the 2014 FIFA World Cup where the Uruguayan player, Álvaro Perreira, was clearly seen to have received a head injury and was rendered unconscious for several seconds, yet on being stretchered off, he returned immediately to the game and continued to play the remaining time (see footage at https://www.youtube.com/watch?v=7OAOX6YnWbU). Fourth, in the NRL, the Parramatta Eels were fined for allowing an apparently concussed player to continue after being assessed by the team doctor. Although the team insisted that the player did not have a concussion, the NRL claimed that the player was returned to the field in such a short time that a thorough concussion assessment could not have taken place.[30]

These 4 cases mark out different ethical concerns with respect to RTP for concussed players. In the first instance, an athletic trainer or health care professional unqualified to make clinical judgments in cases of suspected concussion appraises the status of the player. In the second, the clinical judgment of the sport physician is overruled by the head coach/manager who has no medical qualifications. In the third, the player – whose competence must have been impaired after a concussive episode that appears to last 10 seconds – dictates that he will RTP over the physician's and coach's judgment. In the fourth, irrespective of competence, an unsatisfactory assessment is made and the player returned to the field of play. These cases reveal lacunae in competence, protocol, and compliance.

There have been countless other examples in professional collision sports whereby players have been permitted to RTP despite exhibiting symptoms that indicate concussion (eg, ataxia and brief loss of consciousness), raising questions about undue influence over clinical judgment. Rightly or wrongly, clinicians face questions over their commitment to player welfare in such instances. It is known that team doctors have a conflict of interest although this in itself does not mean that their clinical judgment has been necessarily compromised; rather, it is the tendency for judgment to be influenced unduly that is a problem. But without ways of managing conflicts of interest, there is little idea when a judgment has been improperly influenced.[31]

AUDITING, RECORDING, REPORTING, AND CONFIDENTIALITY

Progress in the clinical management of concussion cases will develop as a response to several factors, including but not limited to (1) increasing sophistication of basic research, (2) increasing convergence on diagnostic tools and protocols, and (3) better understanding of prevalence. For factors (2) and (3) to develop, there must be agreements on how to catalog head injuries and the development of parameters for audits that allow reliable and valid comparisons within teams and sports and across sports too. One important aspect of this process is the management of issues of confidentiality.

Accurate recording and reporting of concussion and mTBI are critical in the interests of athlete welfare and physician protection. It was note above that how various interested parties may wish to not have injuries recorded or reported. To the extent that this happens, auditing of these injuries is invalidated. Might this desire be ethically grounded? Athletes' health status is typically considered sensitive data and is subject to conditions of confidentiality and protected by legal and moral rights to privacy.

In some leagues, such as the NFL in the United States, players may be contracted to have their personal injury data discussed in public. In Europe this is more likely to breach human rights legislation. Notwithstanding, the prevalence of public discussions of such private data, especially in football (soccer) leagues, such as the UK Premiership, is rife.[32,33] Unquestionably, this problem is exacerbated by social media[34] and the use by health care personnel of chat rooms where there is limited protection for the identity of players whose injuries are discussed. Given the serious restrictions that are discussed on safe RTP, athletes will increasingly have an interest in their private data remaining private.

Precisely how data concerning head injuries may be aired is something athletes must be educated in to give their consent. Sports medicine, like many other branches of medicine, is a team affair and athletes must know that for the best care to be given such data must be shared with the rest of the health care team.[35] A recent article by Thompson[36] outlining what might be best practice in terms of appropriate medical oversight and reporting at Princeton University in collegiate sports notes that in many sports no physician is present; while in some sports a physician is present only where available; but that a physician presence is compulsory at a restricted number of targeted sports (eg, at home male football and ice hockey events). At those games where no physician is in attendance and where records are not kept, how will the other members of the sports medical team know if an injury is a repeat one, let alone diagnosed correctly?

Some sports have taken to mandating the reporting of concussion episodes, and this seems to be a crucial measure for understanding the extent of the issue. The Rugby League (United Kingdom) has mandated reporting in all professional games. But it is unclear how the resultant data are stored, accessed, and recorded – whether identifying characteristics have been removed and so on. These are important steps in protecting athletes' best interests. The NFL, for example, receives and stores data centrally by a private company and makes them available for secondary research purposes after appropriate institutional review board approval through the Mount Sinai Hospital in New York. The question arises as to who may legitimately access such data. One point worthy of further professional dialogue and consensus is whether private insurers should be granted access or whether the data should fully be disclosed in any precontract screening if, for example, a college player is drafted into a professional league, a professional player is seeking a transfer to another club, or even if a player is extending a contract.

MATCH DAY DOCTORS: AN INDEPENDENT SOLUTION TO CONFLICTS OF INTEREST AMONG TEAM DOCTORS?

The new NFL protocol requires that an independent neurologic consultant make judgements regarding safe RTP after a concussive episode. This allows for a measure of independence in making this important decision after a positive diagnosis of concussion and initial management. What of the independence of the diagnosis itself though? Some sports leagues have attempted to manage the conflicts of interest faced by team doctors by appointing independent doctors or MDDs to oversee concussion management. A prominent example is the international rugby union tournament between the elite clubs of Australia, New Zealand, and South Africa, known as the Super Rugby or Super 15 competition. Team doctors are still present, but an MDD serves to oversee concussion management and provide additional medical support if required. The rationale for independent MDDs is that because they are not affiliated with any particular team they are shielded from attempts by coaches and players to influence their clinical judgment. MDDs may operate in several roles that could reduce conflicts of interest, although as a novel initiative evidence must be sought to confirm this. First, they may serve as a concussion scouts for both teams in helping to identify suspected concussions that require further assessment. When an MDD sees a player from either side exhibiting concussion symptoms, the MDD could immediately refer the player to the relevant team doctor for assessment. MDDs may also work with video technology to confirm potential incidents or to be informed on incidents that they may have missed. This could conceivably work to relieve the potential excuse that a suspected concussion was not seen by the team doctor and thus not assessed by the team doctor. Secondly, when a suspected concussion is identified, MDDs act as impartial observers of the team doctor's assessment (and diagnosis) or can be asked to conduct the concussion assessment. This may also work to relieve suspicions that concussion assessments are not sufficiently robust or that players have been prematurely passed fit to RTP.

There may also be several practical advantages to having MDDs. Although team doctors are competent and qualified to diagnose concussion, they are not always specialists in concussion. MDDs could be recruited specifically to provide that expertise. In addition, because team doctors are responsible for all the medical needs of an entire team, their attention may be spread across multiple injuries to several players. In free-flowing sports, such as rugby union, this can present a significant challenge and it is not difficult to see how the immediate symptoms of a concussion could be missed by a team doctor attending to the needs of another player.

Despite these potential advantages and the example of their use in the Super 15, proposals to utilize MDDs have not always enjoyed support and their implementation across (and within) sports is patchy. In the NRL, MDDs have been introduced for State of Origin representative matches but not regular season matches, whereas the Australian Football League does not currently have MDDs. The most common argument against widespread implementation in these 2 leagues seems to be the extra cost of employing MDDs to oversee every match; however, there also seem to be clinical concerns. Perhaps team doctors know the players better and might be in a better position to accurately assess a suspected concussion given their knowledge of a player's medical history and baseline testing. Perhaps team doctors may even be more conservative than MDDs – if, for example, the team doctor knows a player has a long history of concussion compared with an MDD who is naïve to such a history. But even if this argument is accepted, it does not seem to negate the use of MDDs to help identify suspected concussions and provide a second opinion on assessment as a way of reducing suspicions of partiality.

SUMMARY

Compared with many other branches of sports medicine, concussion diagnosis and management science and clinical practice are in their early stages of development. The complexity of the neurologic conditions and the lack of consensus over them compound this observation. Although leading concussion experts have identified what they take to be best practice, numerous problems remain in its implementation across the sports spectrum. This article focuses on elite and professional sports, using examples where head contact and injury are likely to be frequent and foreseeable. A range of ethical considerations is identified as they arise in concussion diagnosis and management, including coercion or duress that physicians may face, athlete confidentiality and best interests, and conflicts of interest. Although these problems may arise across the sports spectrum, they will be amplified in the high stakes of certain elite and professional sports. One potential solution is proposed, the use of independent MDDs, which would ameliorate some but not all of these concerns and could be implemented in professional sports with relative ease given a more robust commitment to athlete welfare and sport physician protection.

ACKNOWLEDGMENTS

The authors are most grateful to Richard Lawrance, Kirsten Millen, and Matt Perry for their helpful comments.

REFERENCES

1. Harmon KG, Drezner JA, Gammons M, et al. American Medical Society for Sports Medicine position statement: concussion in sport. Br J Sports Med 2013;47(1): 15–26.
2. Giza CC, Kutcher JS, Ashwal S, et al. Summary of evidence-based guideline update: evaluation and management of concussion in sports: report of the Guideline Development Subcommittee of the American Academy of Neurology. Neurology 2013;80(24):2250–7.
3. Aubry M, Cantu R, Dvorak J, et al. Summary and agreement statement of the first International Conference on Concussion in Sport, Vienna 2001. Br J Sports Med 2002;36(1):6–7.
4. McCrory P, Johnston KM, Meeuwisse W, et al. Summary and agreement statement of the 2nd International Conference on Concussion in Sport, Prague 2004. Br J Sports Med 2005;39(4):196–204.
5. McCrory P, Meeuwisse W, Johnston KM, et al. Consensus Statement on Concussion in Sport: the 3rd International Conference on Concussion in Sport held in Zurich, November 2008. Br J Sports Med 2009;43(Suppl 1):i76–84.
6. McCrory P, Meeuwisse WH, Aubry M, et al. Consensus statement on concussion in sport: the 4th International Conference on Concussion in Sport held in Zurich, November 2012. Br J Sports Med 2013;47(5):250–8.
7. McNamee MJ, Partridge B, Anderson L. Concussion in sport: conceptual and ethical issues. Kinesiol Rev 2015;4(2):190–202.
8. Partridge B. Dazed and confused: sports medicine, conflicts of interest, and concussion management. J Bioeth Inq 2014;11(1):65–74.
9. Partridge B, Hall W. Conflicts of interest in recommendations to use computerized neuropsychological tests to manage concussion in professional football codes. Neuroethics 2014;7(1):63–74.
10. Partridge B. Hit and miss: ethical issues in the implementation of a "concussion rule" in Australian football. AJOB Neurosci 2011;2(4):62–3.
11. Vagnozzi R, Signoretti S, Cristofori L, et al. Assessment of metabolic brain damage and recovery following mild traumatic brain injury: a multicentre, proton magnetic resonance spectroscopic study in concussed patients. Brain 2010;133(11): 3232–42.
12. Vagnozzi R, Signoretti S, Tavazzi B, et al. Hypothesis of the postconcussive vulnerable brain: experimental evidence of its metabolic occurrence. Neurosurgery 2005;57(1):164–71 [discussion: 164–71].
13. Vagnozzi R, Signoretti S, Tavazzi B, et al. Temporal window of metabolic brain vulnerability to concussion: a pilot 1H-magnetic resonance spectroscopic study in concussed athletes–part III. Neurosurgery 2008;62(6):1286–95 [discussion: 1295–6].
14. McKee AC, Stein TD, Nowinski CJ, et al. The spectrum of disease in chronic traumatic encephalopathy. Brain 2013;136:43–64.
15. McNamee M, Partridge B. Concussion in sports medicine ethics: policy, epistemic and ethical problems. Am J Bioeth 2013;13(10):15–7.
16. Valovich McLeod TC, Schwartz C, Bay RC. Sport-related concussion misunderstandings among youth coaches. Clin J Sport Med 2007;17(2):140–2.
17. Malcolm D. Medical uncertainty and clinician-athlete relations: The management of concussion injuries in rugby union. Sociol Sport J 2009;26(2):191–210.
18. Holm S, McNamee M. Ethics in sports medicine. BMJ 2009;339:b3898.
19. Anderson LC, Gerrard DF. Ethical issues concerning New Zealand sports doctors. J Med Ethics 2005;31(2):88–92.

20. Dunn WR, George MS, Churchill L, et al. Ethics in sports medicine. Am J Sports Med 2007;35(5):840–4.
21. Williamson IJ, Goodman D. Converging evidence for the under-reporting of concussions in youth ice hockey. Br J Sports Med 2006;40(2):128–32 [discussion: 128–32].
22. Miyashita TL, Diakogeorgiou E, Hellstrom B, et al. High School Athletes' Perceptions of Concussion. Orthop J Sports Med 2014;2(11):1–5.
23. Meehan WP 3rd, Bachur RG. Sport-related concussion. Pediatrics 2009;123(1): 114–23.
24. Academies, I.o.M.o.t.N. Sports-Related Concussions in Youth Improving the Science, Changing the Culture. 2013. Available at: http://iom.nationalacademies.org/~/media/Files/Report%20Files/2013/Concussions/concussions-RB.pdf.
25. Kroshus E, Garnett B, Hawrilenko M, et al. Concussion under-reporting and pressure from coaches, teammates, fans, and parents. Soc Sci Med 2015;134:66–75.
26. Kroshus E, Baugh CM, Daneshvar DH, et al. Pressure on sports medicine clinicians to prematurely return collegiate athletes to play after concussion. J Athl Train 2015; 50(9):944–51.
27. Orchard J. Concussion: how do we reconcile risk-averse policies with risk-taking sports? In: Khan K, editor. BJSM Blog. 2012. Available at: http://blogs.bmj.com/bjsm/2012/03/15/concussion-how-do-we-reconcile-risk-averse-policies-with-risk-taking-sports/.
28. Crawley P. Wests Tigers hit with $20k concussion fine, but Bulldogs escape punishment. 2014. Available at: http://www.dailytelegraph.com.au/sport/nrl/wests-tigers-hit-with-20k-concussion-fine-but-bulldogs-escape-punishment/story-fni3gpz1-1226909478577. Accessed August 7, 2015.
29. Khan K. Sorry Mr Villas-Boas. "Concussion call ALWAYS belongs to Doctor." BJSM Blog. 2013. Available at: http://blogs.bmj.com/bjsm/2013/11/04/sorry-mr-villas-boas-concussion-call-always-belongs-to-doctor/. Accessed August 7, 2015.
30. Chammas M. Parramatta Eels concede they didn't follow protocol over Nathan Peats concussion but insist he was fit to return. 2015. Available at: http://www.smh.com.au/rugby-league/parramatta-eels/parramatta-eels-concede-they-didnt-follow-protocol-over-nathan-peats-concussion-but-insist-he-was-fit-to-return-20150330-1mb6tg.html#ixzz3i5nuqg3M. Accessed August 7, 2015.
31. Davis M, Stark A, editors. Conflict of interest in the professions. New York: Oxford; 2001.
32. Waddington I, Roderick M. Management of medical confidentiality in English professional football clubs: some ethical problems and issues. Br J Sports Med 2002;36(2):118–23.
33. Ribbans B, Ribbans H, Nightingale C, et al. Sports medicine, confidentiality and the press. Br J Sports Med 2013;47(1):40–3.
34. Olson DE. Team physician challenges in 2013: dealing with media and travelling across state borders. Br J Sports Med 2013;47(1):5–6.
35. Anderson L. Contractual obligations and the sharing of confidential health information in sport. J Med Ethics 2008;34(9):e6.
36. Thompson C. Determining the appropriate model for concussion in health care in college or university setting. Kinesiol Rev 2015;4(2):203–14.

Rethinking the Standard of Care in Treating Professional Athletes

Caroline Poma, BA[a,b], Seth L. Sherman, MD[c], Bradley Spence, BA[d],
Lawrence H. Brenner, JD[e], B. Sonny Bal, MD, JD, MBA[c,]*

KEYWORDS

- Standard of care • Professional athlete • Sports medicine

KEY POINTS

- There is debate over the standard of care that should apply to the medical care of a professional athlete.
- Team physicians are faced with conflicting demands when taking care of professional athletes.
- This article proposes that 1 standard of medical care should apply to all patients.
- The system should adopt a policy that facilitates competitive sports participation, while minimizing the risk of long-term injury.

INTRODUCTION

There has been much public discussion and debate within the medical community about the role of team physicians in professional sports. One law review article, for example, titled "Professional Team Doctors: Money, Prestige, and Ethical Dilemmas," has highlighted the unresolved issues that arise in the relationship between the team doctor and professional sports athletes. The "win at all costs" mentality in professional sports can compromise the team physician's Hippocratic Oath, and create conflicts that can undermine a player's health. Well-recognized team physicians can be helpful in promoting the team brand, such that a team physician may feel a greater sense of allegiance toward the team owners rather than the players.[1]

The previously described observations were captured in a 2013 *Washington Post* survey in which National Football League (NFL) retirees were queried about their

[a] University of North Carolina School of Law, Chapel Hill, NC, USA; [b] University of Virginia, Charlottesville, VA, USA; [c] Department of Orthopedic Surgery, University of Missouri, Columbia, MO, USA; [d] University of Missouri School of Medicine, Columbia, MO, USA; [e] Department of Orthopaedics and Rehabilitation, Yale University, New Haven, CT, USA
* Corresponding author. Missouri Orthopaedic Institute, 1100 Virginia Avenue, DC953.00, Columbia, MO 65212.
E-mail address: balb@health.missouri.edu

Clin Sports Med 35 (2016) 269–274
http://dx.doi.org/10.1016/j.csm.2015.10.001
0278-5919/16/$ – see front matter © 2016 Elsevier Inc. All rights reserved.

perception of team physician priorities. Only 13% perceived that their health was the team physician's priority, while 47% responded that the team physician's priority was the interest of the team itself.[2] Injured athletes can place pressure on team physicians to prematurely return them to play, because of financial rewards, an aggressive, sports-driven environment, and worries that a substitute player could replace the injured player. The team physician is thus caught in a dual and sometimes competing obligation to the player and the team. The obligation to players is to protect the player from further injury, while the obligation to the team is to win, even if winning risks the premature return of an injured player to the field. In contrast, the standard of care that ordinary physicians recognize is driven by the sole aim of ensuring patient well-being and health.

In an effort to eliminate the conflicts that sports team physicians may encounter, some authors have suggested that the role of the team physician should be eliminated entirely.[3] However, physicians can face similar conflicts in other roles as well. Thus, similar to team physicians, the so-called company doctors who are employed by corporations can also face a dual obligation (ie, an obligation to ensure the employee–patient's welfare, vs looking out for the company's financial health, and a desire to maximize worker productivity). Likewise, worker compensation physicians may face a conflict when treating an injured patient (ie, financial pressures that urge a quick return to work at the least cost vs treating the patient covered by a worker compensation claim just as any other patient).

To facilitate the care of patients covered by worker compensation claims, many states have established guidelines through boards and related bodies that specify the standard of care that should apply. In medical negligence claims related to treatments rendered by company doctors, or those rendered by physicians treating worker compensation patients, courts have used the generally accepted standard to care that applies to medical practice. The reason that professional sports team physicians are different is the high public profile of national teams, intense media coverage, the competitive nature of professional sports, large financial considerations, the need to expedite medical decisions in the heat of the moment, and the enormous impact of those decisions on the outcome for the team owners and players. Additionally, sports team physicians often have a variety of financial relationships with the team owners, leading to additional factors that impinge upon medical decision making in the professional sports setting.[4]

Overall, physicians serving professional sports teams are confronted with conflicting demands, in terms of prioritizing the health of the patient–athlete, versus looking out for the team interest in a highly competitive, publicly visible, and financially rewarding environment. Ordinarily, 1 standard of care applies to medical care (ie, the physician must protect and maximize patient welfare over all other considerations). The dilemma facing team physicians challenges this simple assumption, and some authors have suggested that a different standard of medical care should apply to team physicians. This article proposes instead that a single standard—consistent with the Hippocratic Oath—can suffice and address the interests of all stakeholders.

ATHLETIC INJURIES AND A POLICY PROPOSAL

As the role and obligations of team physicians continues to be debated, public awareness about the devastating impact of professional sports activities, such as football, has increased. Public awareness has been driven, at least in part, by litigation initiated by retired players against the NFL, along with media reports suggesting that the NFL withheld data about the long-term consequences of sports injuries,[5] and increasing awareness of the incidence of concussions and the sequelae of devastating physical injuries among retired professionals.[2]

The starting point for any discussion about the standards of care for team physicians needs to begin with a health policy statement. This article sets forth the proposition that team physicians, through their professional associations, should develop a health policy. The policy would specify that after a professional athlete has completed a sports career, his or her cognitive and physical health should not be so compromised that future quality of life is affected. This health policy statement provides a framework for resolving the conflicts that team physicians can face in providing care to professional athletes.

An advantage of this policy is that it is entirely consistent with a physician's obligation as embodied in the Hippocratic Oath. Although it is easy enough to agree with the general policy statement offered, it will inevitably raise questions among sports fans, team owners, coaches, and players. These questions include:

1. Would such a health policy reduce the playing time of all players?
2. Would such a policy fundamentally change the highly competitive and aggressive nature of certain sports, such as professional football?
3. Should a professional player be permitted to consent to substandard care in the interest of expediting return to the field?

These questions are relevant in the competitive and financially lucrative field of professional sports. Stakeholders, such as the team ownership, fan base, and the players, may prefer to perpetuate the status quo instead, with only minor changes to the management and treatment of player's cognitive and physical injuries. In order to ensure that team physicians do not face conflicting demands, and provide care that is consistent with accepted standards of care, the authors propose adoption of the following principles:

1. *The professional athlete should receive the same standard of care as that received by the general public.* There is an unresolved issue of whether there should be a different (and perhaps lesser) standard of care for team physicians, than physicians providing care to nonprofessional athletes. Such a bifurcated standard of care is inconsistent with the role of a physician whose obligation is to provide a consistent level and quality of patient care, regardless of the environment. To bifurcate this standard and accept that there is one standard for professional athletes and a different one for the general public, introduces into the physician–patient relationship factors that may be inconsistent with the goal of protecting the health and well-being of the patient.

The legal cases that have addressed the appropriate standard of care for team physicians treating professional athletes are limited in terms of their ability to help resolve the issue of what standard, or standards of care, should apply to the care of professional athletes. In a legal ruling titled *Zimbauer v. Milwaukee Orthopedic Group*, the court dismissed a pitcher's claim for injuries that were inappropriately treated on the grounds that the expert witness for the injured athlete failed to establish an appropriate sports medicine standard of care.[6] The court appears to have accepted, at face value, the assumption that there was a different standard of care to be provided to a professional athlete as opposed to the general public. The court was unable to clearly express a rationale for a separate standard or articulate what that standard should be.

The importance of a single standard of medical care was illustrated in another legal case titled *Bill Walton v. The Portland Trail Blazers*. This litigation was settled out of court, and no written opinion was ever issued, thus limiting the precedential value of this lawsuit.[7] Bill Walton, a star professional basketball player, sued the Portland Trail

Blazers team doctors, alleging that a foot fracture would not have occurred but for narcotic injections that numbed his pain. The suit alleged that the team physician did not warn Walton of the risks of these pain-killing injections, which included career-ending permanent injuries. The facts showed that the same symptoms would have been treated differently in a nonathlete, with conservative care, such as a protective device and activity modification.

The *Walton* case shows that pain is treated differently in professional athletes who are in the midst of sports participation, versus routine patients. In a professional sports setting, pain is often masked, and considerations of full recovery are postponed until season end. In nonathletes, pain may result in immobilization and activity restriction, with return to full function delayed or limited until full recovery. A single standard of care for athletes and nonathletes alike would resolve the conflicts that face team physicians, allowing the delivery of objective and appropriate care to the athlete.

2. *A single standard of care may encourage important changes that improve the health and well-being of the players.* If team physicians embraced a single standard of care, then professional sports associations, such as the NFL, would adapt accordingly. One such adaptation could be an expansion of the team roster. By expanding the team roster, there would be less competitive pressure for an injured player to return to the game prematurely. Such an expansion may also help to redefine what a starting position is in the NFL. Clarification of the starting position through an expanded roster may have avoided the injury that occurred, for example, in the highly publicized case of Washington Redskins Quarterback Robert Griffin III.

In the 2013 NFL playoffs, Griffin, popularly known as RG3, suffered a knee injury.[8] After he was briefly examined by team physicians, he persuaded the coach to let him back on the field, asserting that he was experiencing pain but had not suffered an injury. RG3 lacked the medical knowledge to make such a decision, and the coaches should have recognized that he lacked such expertise. He returned to the field with the approval of the coaches and team physicians; these decisions were undoubtedly influenced by the desire to see the team win. By the fourth quarter, his condition and playing ability had deteriorated, and he suffered a torn ligament in his right knee.[8]

This particular case may represent what happens to players when they are under duress and acting in the heat of the moment. They may be incapable of thoughtfully thinking through the impact that their injury may have on their long-term health and well-being, given the acute urgency that they return to the game. Such a sense of urgency precludes a thoughtful discussion with the team physician about whether a return to the game represents an unacceptable health risk to the player. Under the model proposed, the standard of care for a team physician would be to thoroughly evaluate the player, even though time may be of the essence from the standpoint of the team winning or losing a game. More important, the team physician, and not the player, would communicate to the training staff and/or coach regarding the player's status. To comply with the standard of care, the team physician's decision would have to be dissociated from any consideration of what the game status was, or whether it was a regular-season or postseason game. Another option may be to modify the rules of the game to assist in achieving the proposed health policy. It may be something as simple as more strictly redefining unnecessary roughness. Football will always be a rough contact sport, but the object is to make it safer with less risk of long-term damage to the players.

3. *It would be below the standard of care for a physician to acquiesce to a player's desire to re-enter a game when return to sports risks further harm.* One of the questions raised previously is the role of the team physician when the player consents to

treatment below the standard of care. The most common example of this is a player's desire to prematurely return to active participation when such active participation is not in the player's best health interest. If a physician agrees to allow the player to return even though he or she holds the opinion that such return presents an unreasonable risk of harm to the player, the law should hold that the physician has violated the standard of care. Moreover, if the player returns, and the physician does not notify the team that his return is against medical advice, the team physician has violated the standard of care. Finally, the decision on whether a patient should return to the game should be no different than what a physician would advise a patient in a routine, nonathletic setting.

SUMMARY

A physician has a professional and legal duty to provide care to patients that is consistent with the standard of care. This obligation is universally recognized by all physicians, regardless of their specialty, and has withstood the test of time. The issue of whether that obligation applies equally in the care of professional athletes where competitive and financial pressures may present intense conflicts has been debated, without a clear resolution. Although the team owners, coaches, and professional players themselves may have a variety of interests that supersede considerations for the player's health, those interests should play no role in the physician–patient relationship. The team physician's obligation is to operate within the generally accepted standard of medical care even if the patient is a professional athlete, and the law should recognize this obligation.

To place the previously described principle into practice, it would be useful for professional associations of team physicians to establish a health policy statement such as the one suggested within this article. One of the most important aspects of a team physician operating within the standard of care is to prevent injury, rather than react to such after it has occurred. Although such a health policy may require adaptations by the team, these adaptations should be of no concern to the team physician. As Sally Jenkins and Rick Maese observed in a 2013 *Washington Post* article, "There is medicine, and then there is NFL medicine, and the practice of the two isn't always the same."[9] Under a single standard of care model, there will only be the practice of medicine, regardless of the patient's occupation. A single standard of care will ensure the long-term safety and well-being of athlete–patients, minimize conflicts for team physicians, and enhance the public view of physician independence and professionalism.

REFERENCES

1. Caldarone JP. Professional team doctors: money, prestige, and ethical dilemmas. Sports Law J 2002;9:131–51.
2. NFL retirees happy with football career despite lasting pain. The Washington Post. Available at: http://www.washingtonpost.com/page/2010-2019/WashingtonPost/2013/05/17/National-Politics/Polling/release_236.xml. Accessed July 30, 2015.
3. Bal SB, Brenner LH. Care of the professional athlete: what standard of care? Clin Orthop Relat Res 2013;471(1):2060–4.
4. Calandrillo SP. Sports medicine conflicts: team physicians vs. athlete–patients. SLU Law J 2006;50:187–209.
5. League of denial: the NFL's concussion crisis. Frontline 2013.
6. Zimbauer v Milwaukee Orthopaedic Group, Ltd. 920 F.Supp. 959 (ED Wis 1996).

7. Walton in Settlement. The New York Times. Available at: http://www.nytimes.com/1982/06/05/sports/walton-in-settlement.html. Accessed July 30, 2015.
8. Shenin D, Maske M, Jones M. Robert Griffin III knee injury: what really led to it during the Redskins-Seahawks game? The Washington Post. Available at: http://www.washingtonpost.com/sports/redskins/robert-griffin-iii-knee-injury-what-really-led-to-it-during-the-redskins-seahawks-game/2013/01/18/752da310-617d-11e2-8f16-7b37a1341b04_story.html. Accessed July 30, 2015.
9. Jenkins S, Maese R. NFL medical standards, practices are different than almost anywhere else. The Washington Post. Available at: http://articles.washingtonpost.com/2013-03-16/sports/37767707_1_robert-griffin-nfl-network-doctors. Accessed July 28, 2015.

Understanding Eating Disorders in Elite Gymnastics

Ethical and Conceptual Challenges

Jacinta Oon Ai Tan, MBBS, MA, MRCPsych, DPhil, MSc[a],*,
Raff Calitri, MSc, PhD[b], Andrew Bloodworth, BSc, PhD[c],
Michael J. McNamee, BA, MA, MA, PhD[d]

KEYWORDS

- Gymnastics • Eating disorders • Depressive symptoms • Self-esteem
- Female athlete triad syndrome • Elite performance

KEY POINTS

- Symptoms of eating disorders are more prevalent in high performance gymnasts than the normal population.
- The definition of eating disorders is problematic when applied to the high performance gymnastics environment.
- The high levels of eating disordered attitudes and behaviors and depressive and anxiety symptoms should be of concern, especially given the young age of this population.

INTRODUCTION

Eating disorders are serious mental disorders characterized by an overvalued desire to lose weight and/or be thin or a fear of fatness, a distorted body image, and associated behaviors.[1] They tend to begin in adolescence and young adulthood, and can derail development and life courses.[2,3] The mortality associated with eating disorders is the highest of all mental disorders, with deaths occurring not only in the throes of severe disorder but even years afterward, both owing to suicide and the physical consequences of disordered eating and weight loss behaviors.[4–6]

[a] Institute of Life Sciences 2, College of Medicine, Swansea University, Room 306, Floor 3, Singleton Campus, Swansea SA2 8PP, UK; [b] Psychology Applied to Health, College House, University of Exeter Medical School, St. Luke's Campus, Magdalen Road, Exeter EX1 2LU, UK; [c] Interprofessional Studies, College of Human and Health Sciences, Floor 7, Vivian Tower, Swansea University Singleton Campus, Swansea SA2 8PP, UK; [d] College of Engineering, Swansea University Bay Campus, Fabian Way, Swansea SA1 8EN, UK
* Corresponding author.
E-mail address: j.o.a.tan@swansea.ac.uk

Clin Sports Med 35 (2016) 275–292
http://dx.doi.org/10.1016/j.csm.2015.10.002
0278-5919/16/$ – see front matter © 2016 Elsevier Inc. All rights reserved.

Of those who survive, much greater numbers suffer from psychiatric comorbidities and physical disabilities such as cardiac problems, gastrointestinal problems, osteoporosis, infertility, and neurologic deficits; some of these irreversible.[7] Treatments for eating disorders are often ineffective and a majority of sufferers either remain chronically unwell or suffer a relapsing and remitting course.[2] The best outcomes for eating disorders are seen when eating disorders are detected early in younger individuals and prompt treatment is provided to prevent them from becoming entrenched or chronic.[8,9] The cost of eating disorders to individuals, families, and society in terms of suffering, loss of potential and treatment costs are immense.[10] The prevention, early identification, and treatment of eating disorders are therefore of paramount importance.[9–11]

It is well-established that eating disorders have a greater prevalence among elite and high performance sport as compared with the normal population, with a particularly high prevalence in disciplines that emphasize leanness, low weight, or (slim) aesthetics.[12,13] The term female athlete triad was coined to characterize a variant of eating disorders commonly found in female athletes, consisting of disordered eating, menstrual dysfunction, and low bone mass.[14,15] Research has investigated the characteristics of eating disorders and the female athlete triad among athletes, and also the effects of high levels of physical training on the growth and sexual development of girls and young women.[14,16]

Despite considerable scientific research, some conceptual issues in the context of eating disorders and elite sports remain largely unaddressed. Research studies largely assume that mental health criteria developed for the normal population can be applied to the high performance sports domain.[12] This assumption, however, that mental health criteria and concepts map well onto the particular and unusual context of high performance sports is problematic. In the process of conducting our empirical research, it became clear that there are difficulties with operating the current definition of eating disorders in an elite sport environment, where some features common to eating disorders are normalized within that milieu.[17] Herein we report on a quantitative and qualitative study into disordered eating and eating disorders, in which a range of conceptual and ethical difficulties raised clear problems for research, diagnosis, and treatment.[17]

EATING DISORDERS: CLASSIFICATION AND DIAGNOSIS

There are 3 main eating disorders, namely, anorexia nervosa, bulimia nervosa, and binge eating disorder.[18] Binge eating disorder is a recently recognized diagnosis in the newly released *Diagnostic and Statistical Manual of Mental Disorders* (DSM)-5 (the American Psychiatric Association's Diagnostic Classification system) and is mostly associated with obesity.[18] In addition to individuals who fulfill criteria for these specific eating disorders, there are greater numbers who are significantly eating disordered but do not fulfill criteria; these are variously classified as eating disorder not otherwise specified in the *International Classification of Diseases* (ICD)-10 (which is the World Health Organization's classification of psychiatric disorders),[19,20] or other specified feeding or eating disorder and unspecified feeding or eating disorder in the DSM-5.[21]

Eating disorders are characterized generally by disordered eating behaviors and distorted cognitions concerning food, weight, and shape. In anorexia nervosa, there is a strong drive to be thin or lose weight with self-induced weight loss, which is associated with distorted body perception and self-image; in bulimia nervosa, there are cycles of bingeing and purging that are associated with similar cognitive distortions. **Boxes 1** and **2** provide the current ICD-10 criteria for anorexia nervosa and bulimia nervosa, respectively, and **Box 3** provides a list of the other ICD-10 and DSM-5 eating disorders.

Box 1
Diagnostic criteria for anorexia nervosa

ICD-10: F50.0 Anorexia nervosa

A. Weight loss, or in children a lack of weight gain, leading to a body weight of at least 15% below the normal or expected weight for age and height.

B. The weight loss is self-induced by avoidance of "fattening foods."

C. A self-perception of being too fat, with an intrusive dread of fatness, which leads to a self-imposed low weight threshold.

D. A widespread endocrine disorder involving the hypothalamic–pituitary–gonadal axis, manifest in the female as amenorrhea, and in the male as a loss of sexual interest and potency (an apparent exception is the persistence of vaginal bleeds in anorexic women who are on replacement hormonal therapy, most commonly taken as a contraceptive pill).

E. Does not meet criteria A and B of bulimia nervosa (F50.2).

Comments (in ICD-10):
The following features support the diagnosis, but are not necessary elements: self-induced vomiting; self-induced purging; excessive exercise; use of appetite suppressants and/or diuretics.
If onset is prepubertal, the sequence of pubertal events is delayed or even arrested (growth ceases; in girls the breasts do not develop and there is a primary amenorrhea; in boys the genitals remain juvenile). With recovery, puberty is often completed normally, but the menarche is late.

Adapted from World Health Organization. International Statistical Classification of Diseases and Related Health Problems, 10th Revision (ICD-10). Geneva: WHO, 1992.

Eating disorders tend to emerge in adolescence and young adulthood. Anorexia nervosa has a typical onset at 13 to 19 years, whereas bulimia nervosa has a slightly older typical age of onset.[5] Females are at greater risk of developing eating disorders, although males can suffer from them as well.[22] Risk factors for eating disorders

---

Box 2
Diagnostic criteria for bulimia nervosa

ICD 10: F50.2 Bulimia nervosa

A. Recurrent episodes of overeating ($\geq$2 times per week over a period of 3 months) in which large amounts of food are consumed in short periods of time.

B. Persistent preoccupation with eating and a strong desire or a sense of compulsion to eat (craving).

C. The patient attempts to counteract the fattening effects of food by 1 or more of the following:
   1. Self-induced vomiting;
   2. Self-induced purging;
   3. Alternating periods of starvation; or
   4. Use of drugs such as appetite suppressants, thyroid preparations or diuretics. When bulimia occurs in diabetic patients they may choose to neglect their insulin treatment.

D. A self-perception of being too fat, with an intrusive dread of fatness (usually leading to underweight).

Adapted from World Health Organization. International Statistical Classification of Diseases and Related Health Problems, 10th Revision (ICD-10). Geneva: WHO, 1992.

Box 3
Other eating disorder diagnoses in ICD-10 and DSM 5

ICD-10:

- F50.1 Atypical anorexia nervosa

- F50.3 Atypical bulimia nervosa

- F50.8 Other eating disorders

- F50.9 Eating disorder, unspecified

DSM-5:

- Binge eating disorder

- Pica

- Rumination disorder

- Avoidant/restrictive food intake disorder (ARFID)

- Other specified feeding or eating disorder (OSFED)

- Purging disorder

- Night eating syndrome

- Unspecified feeding or eating disorder (UFED)

Adapted from World Health Organization. International Statistical Classification of Diseases and Related Health Problems, 10th Revision (ICD-10). Geneva: WHO, 1992; and American Psychiatric Association. Diagnostic and statistical manual of mental disorders. Fifth edition (DSM-5). Arlington (VA): American Psychiatric Association; 2013.

---

include a family history of eating disorders, parental dieting or disordered eating behaviors, and personality traits of perfectionism and obsessionality.[23] Some common triggers for the development of eating disorders are dissatisfaction with body shape and weight (eg, as the body is changing in adolescence), dieting behaviors, traumatic or illness experiences, and bullying.[23] It is well-established that context is important, and cultures and environments that place pressure on individuals to conform to unrealistically thin body ideals place individuals at risk for eating disorders, with the prevalence of eating disorders much higher among ballet dancers and models.[24,25]

There are physical and psychological developmental concerns associated with eating disorders in children and adolescents. When individuals develop eating disorders during adolescence, many of the developmental trajectories can be arrested or derailed because physical height, hormonal changes, and bone growth are affected by nutritional fluctuations and/or deficiencies; social isolation and a narrowing of interests or growing comorbid depression can affect academic and social development at a time when exploration of the social environment, friendships and intellectual capacities are usually increasing; and the young person's development of identity and self-image can also be affected.[10,26,27]

There are continuing conceptual and definitional controversies in eating disorders. The new DSM-5 classification published in 2014 loosened the criteria for both anorexia nervosa and bulimia nervosa to enable more sufferers to be categorized as having these disorders.[21] The rationale behind this was that the majority of people suffering from disordered eating and eating disorders failed to meet criteria for these 2 disorders and were relegated to the ill-defined catch-all 'atypical' and 'eating disorder not otherwise specified' categories, which is unhelpful because these 'atypical' categories are both poorly researched and undertreated.[21] A further difficulty is the shifting course of eating disorders within individuals; it has been shown that the majority of sufferers shift from 1 diagnosis to another in the course of their illness.[28] Proposals of a 'transdiagnostic eating disorders' categorization have been made to reflect the fluctuating nature of many eating disorders.[29] Despite this lack of clarity, distinct differences remain between anorexia nervosa and bulimia nervosa that are relevant to both conceptualization, diagnosis, and treatment.[30,31]

Anorexia nervosa is characterized by weight loss and is particularly distinctive because of its egosyntonic nature; that is, it is often experienced as part of the self or congruent with the person's orientation and desires.[32,33] As a result, even when it is very severe and causing significant harm or debility, sufferers may deny they have an illness and claim their starvation is a matter of personal or lifestyle choice.[34–36] This is exemplified by the 'Pro-Ana' underground subculture, which may glorify anorexia nervosa and individuals trade tips online about how to lose more weight and deceive health professionals, or the subversion of treatment efforts that can occur.[36,37] Even when in distress or suffering from diminishing function and increasing risk, sufferers can often be attached to their disorder or feel deep ambivalence to receiving treatment to the extent that compulsory treatment may be needed to save life.[38,39] Because of the opposing effects of bingeing and purging, bulimia nervosa sufferers may be low, normal, or high in weight, and can more easily escape detection. The bingeing and purging behaviors adopted in bulimia nervosa can nevertheless lead to high risks of physical harm.[7]

THE HIGH PERFORMANCE GYMNASTICS ENVIRONMENT

Gymnasts aspiring to elite level typically enter and peak in the high performance arena at a young age. Specialization and intensive training begins very early in life, and most competitive gymnasts retire before their mid 20s.[40] The time window of peak performance often coincides with adolescence, and these adolescent athletes have to cope with both the demands of a high performance environment and the changes associated with physical and sexual growth and maturation.[41] It is important to understand how these changes are interpreted by gymnasts themselves. These normal developmental changes may be viewed in the gymnastics context as both undesirable and deleterious to performance, as illustrated by this female gymnast.

> But I mean like when we get boobs and bums and hips and, it is, you kind of think, "Well go away for a bit, come back when I'm older, I don't need you now."

Because of their relatively young age and the intensive nature of high performance training required, coaches have extensive contact with high performance gymnasts and become important in providing psychological support and structure to their athletic lives, which spills over into everyday life. Most coaches are in effect acting in loco parentis. In the process of shaping their young protégés' bodies and performance, coaches develop strong bonds of trust and shape their attitudes and values, transmitting their own values and goals to the developing gymnasts.[42] The heteronomous nature of this relationship, and the high levels of external structure normal and necessary to the high performance environment, are accentuated by the nature of the relationship, where the youth of many gymnasts means that there is a dependence and clear asymmetry in power and experience, and the gymnast has to trust his or her coach implicitly to know the athlete's limits and capabilities better than the gymnast himself or herself could.[42]

There is a constant focus on optimizing weight for performance in high performance gymnastics, consistent with any high performance sport; but in gymnastics (depending on discipline), there can be an additional element of the demands of aesthetic judging, which idealizes the slim physique and the constant drive to optimize maximal power and performance for minimal weight.[13,43] There are clear differences between different gymnastics disciplines, in performance and aesthetics demands.[44] Tumbling requires small yet very powerful physiques, with less emphasis on slimness. Rhythmic gymnasts, are typically tall and slim with a uniformity of shape and size across the team. In sport acrobatic gymnasts work in teams, with specific roles. Bases have to be strong and powerful and are usually older whereas the 'tops' have to be small and light and are usually younger.[44] Some disciplines or competition formats require conformity and teamwork so relationships with and responsibilities to teammates become important.[44]

THE RESEARCH STUDY

The aim of the overall study was to study the ethical issues involved in eating disorders, and the aim of the quantitative substudy was to ascertain the pattern of eating disorder symptoms, symptoms of depression and levels of self-esteem among high performance British gymnasts aged 10 to 25 years. Our particular focus herein is on the conceptual and ethical issues in diagnosing eating disorders that became apparent as the study progressed, that the physician should be aware of to support, diagnose, and/or treat adolescent athletes in high-level sports environments.

METHODS

In collaboration with British Gymnastics, coaches of selected high performance gymnastics clubs were invited to facilitate recruitment of the sample. This study was reviewed and approved by the Swansea University Research Ethics Committee. All participants (and their parents if under 18) were given invitation letters, information sheets, and consent forms via their coaches, who also provided access for data collection at their regular training venue in confidential settings. All participants signed consent forms, with additional consent provided by parents of participants aged less than 16 years. Each participant was given a set of 4 self-administered questionnaires and then interviewed individually. Participation in research was followed by a psycho-education session for gymnasts (and separately with parents) about eating disorders. All high performance gymnasts aged 10 to 25 years old training were eligible to take part in this study. Fieldwork took place between November 2011 and March 2012 at 4 high performance clubs across Britain.

Four questionnaires were used: the Eating Attitudes Test (EAT-26),[45] the Eating Disorder Examination Questionnaire Version (EDE-Q6),[46] the Beck Depression Inventory (BDI-II)[47]; and the Rosenberg Self Esteem Scale.[48] The EDE-Q6 is a detailed questionnaire that provides detailed scores on 4 subscales (restraint, eating concern, weight concern, and shape concern)[46]; it has been shown to be an accurate screening tool for identifying likely cases of eating disorders in the community.[49] The EAT-26 is a briefer screening instrument that has been found to be useful in identifying athletes at risk of eating disorders.[50] The Rosenberg Self-Esteem Scale indicates whether there is significant low self-esteem.[48] The BDI differentiates between symptoms of mild, moderate, and severe depression.[47] The EDE-Q6, EAT-26, BDI, and Rosenberg Self-Esteem Scale are all validated for ages 12 and older.[47,48,50–55] The participants' self-reported dates of birth, height, and weight were also collected at the same time.

RESULTS

A total of 51 male (n = 16) and female (n = 35) high performance gymnasts from 4 clubs completed the questionnaire, from the disciplines of tumbling (n = 7), acrobatics (n = 28), and rhythmic gymnastics (n = 16). There were 38 gymnasts were competing at international level and 13 at national level. **Table 1** characterizes the sample and questionnaire scores. Four of these participants were aged younger than 12 years and have been excluded from the analyses that follow because there are no norms for individuals younger than 12 years in the instruments used. The project also involved semistructured interviews with gymnasts and support staff (n = 42). These are only briefly reported on herein; a more detailed analysis of these findings is published.[56]

On the Rosenberg Self-Esteem Scale, 5 athletes (11%) had low self-esteem (<15 indicates low self-esteem). Nine athletes (18%) had scores of greater than 25. On the BDI, 26 (55%) had scores indicating minimal or no depression (range 0–9), 19 (40%) had scores indicative of mild depression (range 10–18), and 3 (6%) had scores suggestive of moderate levels of depression. On the EAT 26, 9 athletes (19%) had scores indicating a significant eating problem (≥20). The EDE-Q6 showed far higher proportions above population norms: 67% of females 16 years or older, 61% of females younger than 16 years, and 31% of males had mean EDE-Q6 global scores above population norms.

Table 2 shows the bivariate correlations between all study variables for all gymnasts. Sex was associated with self-esteem and disordered eating behaviors and

Table 1
Descriptive summary of sample and questionnaire scores

Characteristic	n	Minimum	Maximum	Mean	SD
Age	47	12.14	21.36	16.70	2.46
BMI centile	42	0.07	89.56	41.94	29.15
Rosenberg self-esteem	47	11.00	30.00	20.72	4.57
BDI	47	.00	28.00	8.79	5.54
EAT-26	47	.00	46.00	10.13	10.56
EDE-Q6 global	47	.00	5.35	1.69	1.53
EDE-Q6 restraint	47	.00	5.00	1.69	1.55
EDE-Q6 eating concern	45	.00	5.00	.89	1.24
EDE-Q6 shape concern	47	.00	6.00	2.15	1.87
EDE-Q6 weight concern	47	.00	5.80	1.95	1.84

EDE-Q6 Norms	Male (n = 16)	Female ≥16 (n = 18)	Female <16 (n = 13)
EDE-Q6 global norm (n, % above norm)	0.45 (5, 31)	1.59 (12, 67)	1.5 (8, 61)
EDE-Q6 restraint (n, % above norm)	0.15 (9, 56)	1.29 (14, 78)	1.0 (7, 54)
EDE-Q6 Eating concern norm (n, % above norm)	0.69 (2, 12)	0.87 (7, 39)	2.2 (2, 15)
EDE-Q6 shape concern norm (n, % above norm)	0.48 (6, 37)	2.29 (12, 67)	1.8 (9, 69)
EDE-Q6 weight concern norm (n, % above norm)	0.44 (7, 44)	1.89 (11, 61)	1.6 (8, 61)

Note: EDE-Q6 Male norms are derived from Reas and colleagues,[29] Female ≥16 norms from Mond and colleagues[27]; female <16 norms from Carter and colleagues.[13]

Abbreviations: BDI, Beck depression inventory; BMI, body mass index; EDE, Eating Disorder Examination Questionnaire Version; SD, standard deviation.

Data from Refs.[13,27,29]

Table 2
Bivariate correlation (ns range 44–51)

Variable	1	2	3	4	5	6	7	8	9	10	11
1. Sex	—	—	—	—	—	—	—	—	—	—	—
2. Level of competition	−.04	—	—	—	—	—	—	—	—	—	—
3. Age	.16	−.53[a]	—	—	—	—	—	—	—	—	—
4. BMI centile	.13	−.28[c]	.56[a]	—	—	—	—	—	—	—	—
5. Rosenberg self-esteem	.42[a]	.02	−.06	−.06	—	—	—	—	—	—	—
6. BDI	−.23	−.19	.25[c]	.15	−.52[a]	—	—	—	—	—	—
7. EAT-26	−.39[a]	−.11	−.07	−.05	−.11	.50[a]	—	—	—	—	—
8. EDE-Q6 global	−.53[a]	−.20	.06	−.05	−.21	.55[a]	.80[a]	—	—	—	—
9. EDE-Q6 restraint	−.45[a]	−.31[b]	.21	−.02	−.13	.53[a]	.80[a]	.90[a]	—	—	—
10. EDE-Q6 eating concern	−.39[a]	−.14	−.01	−.13	−.03	.43[a]	.68[a]	.87[a]	.75[a]	—	—
11. EDE-Q6 shape concern	−.53[a]	−.12	.07	−.02	−.34[b]	.56[a]	.74[a]	.96[a]	.81[a]	.77[a]	—
12. EDE-Q6 weight concern	−.45[a]	−.18	.00	−.05	−.23	.51[a]	.78[a]	.96[a]	.83[a]	.77[a]	.93[a]

Abbreviations: BDI, Beck depression inventory; BMI, body mass index; EDE, Eating Disorder Examination Questionnaire Version.
[a] Correlation significant at the 0.01 level (2-tailed).
[b] Correlation significant at the 0.05 level (2-tailed).
[c] Correlation marginally significant at the 0.10 level (2-tailed).

attitudes, with males reporting higher levels of self-esteem than females, and females indicating greater propensity for eating disorder symptoms, particularly in the EDE-Q6 restraint, weight concern, and shape concern subscales. International gymnasts generally reported greater restraint over eating than national gymnasts. Self-esteem was marginally negatively associated with shape concern. Higher levels of self-esteem were linked with fewer concerns about body shape. Depressive symptoms were associated positively with eating disorder symptoms. As expected, all of the eating disorder measures (EAT26 and EDE-Q6, along with all the subcomponents of the EDE-Q6) were highly correlated.

The EDE-Q6 asks 3 questions concerning menstrual status, requiring free responses. The responses were converted into a variable (menstrual status) that was subject to bivariate correlation analysis. **Table 3** shows bivariate analysis for females only. **Table 4** shows male gymnasts' data. In females, menstrual status is highly correlated with the EDE-Q6 global, restraint subscale, and eating concern subscale scores, and significantly correlated with the shape concern subscale, weight concern subscale, and EAT-26 scores. Body mass index centiles were not correlated significantly with either eating disorder symptom scores either for sex or menstrual status. Additionally, a series of sequential multiple regression models were run to assess the unique effects of each of the key variables on the different eating disorder measures (**Table 5**). Specifically, the analyses examined whether sex, level of competition, age, self-esteem, and depressive symptoms independently predicted eating disorders. A separate analysis was performed for EAT-26, EDE-Q6 Global and each subscale scores, and the proportion of variance is also reported.

The patterns of relationships were similar between male and female gymnasts. Self-esteem was independently associated with eating disorder symptoms (restraint and eating concerns subscales) and marginally associated with EAT-26 and EDE-Q6 global measures of eating disorders. An increase in self-esteem was linked to an increase in eating disorder symptoms. However, most of the participants had 'good'

Table 3
Bivariate correlation: female athletes (ns range 22–31)

Variable	1	2	3	4	5	6	7	8	9	10	11
1. Level of competition	—	—	—	—	—	—	—	—	—	—	—
2. Age	-.54[a]	—	—	—	—	—	—	—	—	—	—
3. BMI centile	-.02	.40[b]	—	—	—	—	—	—	—	—	—
4. Rosenberg self-esteem	-.20	-.17	-.12	—	—	—	—	—	—	—	—
5. BDI	-.07	.27	.17	-.13	—	—	—	—	—	—	—
6. EAT-26	-.12	-.04	.01	.28	.44[b]	—	—	—	—	—	—
7. EDE-Q6 global	-.25	.23	.08	.20	.55[a]	.76[a]	—	—	—	—	—
8. EDE-Q6 restraint	-.38[b]	.40[b]	.06	.29	.45[b]	.76[a]	.88[a]	—	—	—	—
9. EDE-Q6 eating concern	-.18	.06	-.05	.34[c]	.43[b]	.67[a]	.87[a]	.73[a]	—	—	—
10. EDE-Q6 shape concern	-.17	.26	-.14	-.03	.61[a]	.69[a]	.95[a]	.74[a]	.75[a]	—	—
11. EDE-Q6 weight concern	-.21	.15	.07	.17	.49[a]	.73[a]	.96[a]	.80[a]	.74[a]	.92[a]	—
12. Menstrual status	-.29	.43[b]	.15	-.01	.04	.44[b]	.50[b]	.60[a]	.53[b]	.45[b]	.43[b]

Note: For the variable menstrual status, analysis was carried on the subgroup of all females (n = 24) who remained after removing individuals who provided information suggesting they definitely or may not have yet achieved menarche; failed to provide (sufficient) information about menstrual status; provided menstrual data that were unclear; or reported ingestion of hormonal medication. The subgroup divided into individuals who did/did not reported missing menstrual periods in the last 4 months.

Abbreviations: BDI, Beck depression inventory; BMI, body mass index; EDE, Eating Disorder Examination Questionnaire Version.

[a] Correlation significant at the 0.01 level (2-tailed).
[b] Correlation significant at the 0.05 level (2-tailed).
[c] Correlation marginally significant at the 0.10 level (2-tailed).

Table 4
Bivariate correlation: male athletes (N = 16)

Variable	1	2	3	4	5	6	7	8	9	10
1. Level of competition	—	—	—	—	—	—	—	—	—	—
2. Age	-.51[b]	—	—	—	—	—	—	—	—	—
3. BMI centile	-.60[b]	.73[a]	—	—	—	—	—	—	—	—
4. Rosenberg self-esteem	.42	-.11	-.13	—	—	—	—	—	—	—
5. BDI	-.40	.36	.22	-.79[a]	—	—	—	—	—	—
6. EAT-26	-.23	.07	.00	-.49	.66[a]	—	—	—	—	—
7. EDE-Q6 global	-.37	.02	-.03	-.51[b]	.71[a]	.75[a]	—	—	—	—
8. EDE-Q6 restraint	-.34	.11	.07	-.37	.68[a]	.81[a]	.93[a]	—	—	—
9. EDE-Q6 eating concern	-.23	-.05	-.26	-.38	.50[b]	.27	.75[a]	.55[b]	—	—
10. EDE-Q6 shape concern	-.36	.08	.05	-.48	.71[a]	.71[a]	.98[a]	.92[a]	.71[a]	—
11. EDE-Q6 weight concern	-.37	-.12	-.06	-.61[b]	.62[b]	.74[a]	.91[a]	.76[a]	.59[b]	.85[a]

Abbreviations: BDI, Beck depression inventory; BMI, body mass index; EDE, Eating Disorder Examination Questionnaire Version.

[a] Correlation significant at the 0.01 level (2-tailed).
[b] Correlation significant at the 0.05 level (2-tailed).

Table 5
Sequential multiple regression analyses: Predicting eating disorder symptoms

Dependent Variable	EAT26 (n = 51)		EDE-Q6 Global (n = 51)		EDE-Q6 Restraint (n = 51)		EDE-Q6 Eating Concern (n = 49)		EDE-Q6 Shape Concern (n = 51)		EDE-Q6 Weight Concern (n = 51)	
Predictors	Beta	t	Beta	t	Beta	t	Beta	t	Beta	t	Beta	t
Rosenberg self-esteem	.35	2.41[b]	.30	2.32[b]	.37	2.79[a]	.44	2.85[a]	.15	1.21	.23	1.58
BDI	.63	4.42[a]	.57	4.52[a]	.56	4.31[a]	.58	3.88[a]	.49	3.99[a]	.52	3.74[a]
Sex	−.36	−2.71[b]	−.52	−4.44[a]	−.49	−4.11[a]	−.41	−2.67[a]	−.57	−5.00[a]	−.46	−3.58[a]
Age	−.23	−1.59	−.06	−.06	.06	.44	−.17	−1.12	.02	.13	−.14	−1.01
Level of competition	−.14	−.98	−.16	−1.27	−.20	−1.63	−.16	−1.10	−.05	−.41	−.18	−1.32
% Variance	.37[a]		.50[a]		.49[a]		.34[a]		.53[a]		.41[a]	

Abbreviations: BDI, Beck depression inventory; EAT26, Eating Attitudes Test; EDE, Eating Disorder Examination Questionnaire Version.
[a] Correlation significant at the 0.01 level (2-tailed).
[b] Correlation significant at the 0.05 level (2-tailed).

self-esteem and this effect may have been being driven by the minority who scored lowly for self-esteem. Depressive symptoms were associated independently with eating disorders, with greater levels of depressive symptoms as scored by the BDI linked with greater severity of symptoms of eating disorders. Each model explained a 'good' proportion of the variance in eating disorders.

DISCUSSION

The results of this study reflect a high prevalence of eating disordered behaviors and attitudes that are found among high performance gymnasts, when defined using standard mental health criteria.[12] Importantly, 31% of male gymnasts also scored highly on the eating disorder scales, which suggests that male gymnasts must not be overlooked as potentially having disordered eating attitudes and behaviors. There were no reports of purging and bulimia nervosa did not seem to be a likely diagnosis in this particular group of gymnasts, which is consistent with the young age of the sample.

There are difficulties, however, in applying standard eating disorder criteria to this group of individuals. Traits such as perfectionism and obsessionality associated with success in an elite sport context have similarities with those found in eating disordered individuals.[57–59] In this context, the high performance gymnastics "job requirements" are the demand for constant surveillance of dietary intake, frequent self-monitoring of weight and shape (amplifying monitoring of weight and shape by coaches), and high levels of concern about any weight gain and in particular concern about gaining fat, all of which would be considered eating disordered in the mental health context. Here a female athlete participant reflects on a stringent and perhaps even disordered attitude toward food, but cites an ability to switch this off.

I mean I didn't eat a lot at all and what I did eat I constantly knew what I was eating for the right reasons. But I always felt like I was hungry, like if I felt like I wanted to eat, I knew I could just eat. Like the minute I finished I just went back into a regular eating plan straightaway. So it never kind of held me back

The challenge here is discriminating between extreme attitudes and behaviors that, although seemingly disordered, are rationalized in the sporting context, and are reflected on and endorsed by the athlete.[56] As above, where individuals with anorexia nervosa experience the condition as a central aspect of their identity, and positively endorse this aspect, it becomes difficult to dissociate the apparently autonomously choosing person from the apparent disorder.[32] Furthermore, it will be not in the interests of the athlete to reveal their eating-related concerns and issues to the coach for fear of deselection, because health-related concerns may dictate removal from the squad on grounds of their duty of care to the athlete.[60–62]

These concerns may be compounded in sports acrobatics where the gymnasts perform in teams, as interdependent units. Indeed, the attitudes of the gymnasts, particularly among females and the "tops" (ie, the performer at the apex of complex moves where they may be executing complex skills on top of the shoulders of 2 or 3 other gymnasts) of both sexes of the acrobatics teams, were that the prepubertal slim figure was highly prized by the athlete and the team, and where otherwise "normal" growth in height and female sexual development in particular was viewed as problematic and challenging. A difficulty in the opposite direction presented itself when assessing the gymnasts' (self-reported) weights and body mass indices. Because of the relatively high body mass indices of all the gymnasts, none of them satisfied the low weight criterion of anorexia nervosa. These data must be understood against a background of research that shows that bone density and lean body mass are higher in elite gymnasts than normal adolescents.[63,64] Our observational data was that some individuals were very clearly thin and pale, whom the coaches were clearly concerned about, and for whom the clinician researchers among the research team suspected that they were suffering from an eating disorder; however, none of these individuals had a body mass index below 17.5 kg/m^2, nor were they willing to disclose any disordered eating behaviors in their interviews. Indeed, these individuals were less forthcoming about disordered eating behaviors and attitudes than their peers.

These difficulties in matching the standard criteria of eating disorders to this special population raises the possibility that the female athlete triad may be a better means of defining athletes as having eating disorders, because it does not rely on any weight criterion or cognitions. Even so, there are difficulties with this for the specific young population under study. Research suggests that the triad does not identify many of the athletes at risk.[65] Menstrual abnormalities are common as a consequence of the negative energy balance, yet this is difficult to assess in this age group who mostly not have reached or established menarche as they begin high levels of training, and who may suffer delayed menarche rather than a more measurable disruption of already established menstrual cycles. Low bone mineralization is also likely to be a particularly late sign of negative energy balance and severe nutritional problems in this group, because gymnastics is a high-impact sport and tends to increase bone density as compared with normal populations.[63,64,66] Some researchers believe that small stature, late menarche, and late physical maturation are selected for by sports such as gymnastics, rather than being the consequence of intensive training.[41] Finally, disordered eating is a problematic concept when the issue is the "job description" of high performing gymnastics reflected in a highly controlled and restricted intake characteristic of anorexia nervosa.

Many gymnasts in the study had a heavy training load (approximately 25–30 hours per week) in addition to their mainstream educational demands. The BDI responses showed no individuals with thoughts of self-harm or suicide, which contrasts very favorably with 20% to 45% of the adolescent population which reports suicidal thoughts.[67,68] Instead, the gymnasts' questionnaire responses reported difficulties going to sleep, and high levels of anxiety and tiredness. In qualitative data many athletes cited a busy life and restrictions on their spare time, while also referring to the gains from participating in sport at this level.

> Erm … the worst is probably all the time it takes, like with training every single night. I wish I did have a little bit more spare time and stuff. But the best is when you're at a competition and then you just go on the floor and then that just … that feeling that you get. And especially if you win the competition, when you're on the podium it just … it's just an amazing feeling. (Female gymnast)

The findings are not straightforward to interpret, and present conceptual difficulties. There are also limitations to our study. Access to elite sports populations for the purposes of non–performance-enhancing research is problematic. Despite a variety of approaches to weighing practices by coaches, it was not within the scope of the study for the authors to conduct any weighing, physical measurements, or clinical assessments, because the study focused on in-depth interviews yet attempted to be minimally disruptive to the gymnasts' busy training schedules and minimally physically intrusive. The formal diagnosis of any mental disorder requires a full clinical interview, which was also beyond the remit of this study. The method of selection meant that the clubs that volunteered to participate could not be assumed to be representative of high performing clubs in general, and there can be no overarching claims of the representativeness of the data of these high performance gymnasts. Nevertheless, the participants were confident, self-motivated, and ambitious young people, a markedly different population from the standard mental health clinic or the standard school. This was borne out by the high self-esteem scores, which we would suggest reflects the high levels of success, public esteem, and validation associated with successful participation in high performance sport.

Given the occupational requirements of being a high performance athlete in a particularly physically demanding sport, one may ask whether the high scores on the eating disorder questionnaires simply a reflection of a (possibly coincidental) similarity of characteristics between eating disordered people and elite athletes, and the high depression scores are simply a reflection of juggling hectic jobs in addition to being in full-time education. Or is this a highly stressed population constantly performing at their limits, and compromised in their mental health with respect to disordered eating, anxiety and depression as a result? As suggested by 1 participant, 1 distinguishing feature of a functional rather than pathologic preoccupation with weight and shape was whether the individual was able to "switch off" this preoccupation when on holiday from training or, indeed, after retirement from competitive sport. A problem, however, that gymnasts pointed out was that, unlike some other international sports, modern competitive gymnastics does not seem to have any particular "off season" when gymnasts can allow themselves to eat at liberty and gain weight before returning to intensive training and conditioning. Enforcing some kind of off season for athlete rest and recovery could be respite from the constant training and self-discipline that might lend itself to loosening of control and more disordered eating, and that respite might also help to discriminate between those who can stop their "anorexic" attitudes and behaviors when it is not needed and those who cannot. A further issue is that even if functional rather than "mentally disordered," the constant preoccupation with weight and constant idealization of an unrealistic shape, particularly at an important developmental period of self-regulation and self-image is likely to have longer term implications for the way these gymnasts conceptualize and view food and their own bodies or indeed their identities, long after they have retired from the sport.[40,69]

Does the prevalence or normalization of such behaviors and attitudes within a sporting discipline imply that these are normal, healthy, or morally acceptable? To what extent can a physician not intimately familiar with the training demands and milieu of elite gymnasts interpret the fine grained judgements about weight and shape that gymnasts and coaches do as part of the normal everyday encounter with their sport?[62] To the extent that the physician is an insider to the norms and values of the population, how will they guard against "going native" – the anthropologists' nightmare of uncritically accepting the norms of a host population? Without wishing to pathologise emotionally healthy and well-functioning athletes, there is a strong argument that exposure to a negative energy balance and constant preoccupation with weight and shape and high levels of tiredness and anxiety cannot be healthy, especially among young developing minds and bodies at a uniquely susceptible time of life. Some research suggests that postretirement release of high performance athletes from the constraints of low caloric intake can lead to rebound and catch-up physical growth and eventual normal adult height and weight, and there is also an argument that these sports may be self-selecting for smaller, leaner, or slower maturing individuals.[41,70] There is, however, currently relatively little evidence concerning the long-term psychological or emotional implications of these practices, although 1 study suggests that gymnasts' eating disorder symptoms do abate somewhat after retirement; this is clearly an area for researchers to explore further.[71]

There are many similarities but also many differences between eating disorders (in particular anorexia nervosa) and high performance gymnastics. Many people with anorexia nervosa are perfectionistic and obsessional; they are also often highly disciplined and self-controlled and able to focus solely on their goal of weight loss, being able to sacrifice other interests and enjoyments to this goal.[72,73] The similarities in personality between high performance athletes and people with anorexia nervosa places this individuals at particular risk of developing an eating disorder; the contextual pressures within the sport to lose weight and idealization and focus on low weight and slim shape compound these risks.[57] There are arguments that high performance gymnasts may self-select both for body type and also ability to exert high levels of discipline and control over their own bodies and over food intake, and therefore may also be self-selected as being more susceptible to eating disorders as opposed to the sport by its nature inducing these disorders.

There are, however, many differences between high performance sport and eating disorders. For the "functional eating disordered" athlete, the attitudes and behaviors around eating and shape are secondary to an overarching goal of improving performance. In psychiatric eating disordered populations, the attitudes and behaviors have no goal other than themselves, or else serve as some maladaptive coping mechanism, for example, in trying to take control of one's own life in the face of abusive situations or a chaotic family background, although overexercise is often used as a tool to achieve control and weight loss.[23] The nonfunctional and ultimately self-defeating nature of eating disorders is the hallmark of all mental disorders, and such individuals continue to perceive themselves as fat and have a drive to lose weight even when their gain or function is diminishing from malnutrition, psychological difficulties, or poor physical health. In contrast, one might expect an athlete with a functional eating disorder to have the power to cease their weight loss behaviors as they tip over from helpful to harmful with regard to performance and competitiveness. The problem, however, is that there is a fine line between functional and pathological eating attitudes and behaviors; indeed, there may be no line at all. Again, the quality of the athlete–physician relationship is crucial in interpreting this phenomenon with validity and care.[62]

Well-known elite athletes have spoken in hindsight of their own struggles with eating disorders.[74] It may be possible that eating disorders may coexist at the same time as a highly successful sporting career if the athlete succeeds in a precarious balancing act of maintaining control over behavior so that it does not (seriously) harm performance; this may correspond with what clinicians recognize as subclinical eating disorders in the normal population. At the same time, it can be argued that something that is functional in nature may nevertheless be pathological both in terms of its harmfulness and its grip over the psyche.

SUMMARY

The conceptual challenge facing researchers and physicians confronted with potential eating disorders in high performing gymnastics is in distinguishing between functional and pathologic eating attitudes and behaviors in high performance sport. This is crucial if we are to identify those mentally ill individuals (including those with subclinical variants) who need prompt and appropriate help to prevent them from coming to harm, without intervening needlessly in the lives of other individuals who are engaging in similar practices out of necessity without any negative psychological consequences. The practical challenge is in understanding what is harmful for athletes, especially young athletes who are still in the process of physical, emotional, and social development, to promote their current and future well-being; and having understood it, to modify the pressures within the sport to promote well-being and prevent harm.

ACKNOWLEDGMENTS

This research was funded by the Economic and Social Research Council, UK. Project title: *Ethical aspects of the impact of eating disorders on elite gymnasts*. Grant number RES-000-22-4021. The authors gratefully acknowledge the assistance of British Gymnastics, and Steve Green in particular.

REFERENCES

1. Morris J. ABC of eating disorders, vol. 169. Oxford (United Kingdom): John Wiley & Sons; 2011.
2. Berkman ND, Lohr KN, Bulik CM. Outcomes of eating disorders: a systematic review of the literature. Int J Eat Disord 2007;40:293–309.
3. Wade TD, Bergin JL, Tiggemann M, et al. Prevalence and long-term course of lifetime eating disorders in an adult Australian twin cohort. Aust N Z J Psychiatry 2006;40(2):121–8.
4. Arcelus J, Michell AJ, Wales J, et al. Mortality rates in patients with anorexia nervosa and other eating disorders: a meta-analysis of 36 studies. Arch Gen Psychiatry 2011;68(7):724–31.
5. Smink FRE, Van Hoeken D, Hoek HW. Epidemiology of eating disorders: incidence, prevalence and mortality rates. Curr Psychiatry Rep 2012;14(4):406–14.
6. Harris EC, Barraclough B. Excess mortality of mental disorder. Br J Psychiatry 1998;173:11–53.
7. Birmingham CL, Treasure J. Medical management of eating disorders, 2nd edition. Cambridge (United Kingdom): Cambridge University Press; 2010.

8. Campbell K, Peebles R. Eating disorders in children and adolescents: state of the art review. Pediatrics 2014;134(3):582–92.

9. Treasure J, Russell G. The case for early intervention in anorexia nervosa: theoretical exploration of maintaining factors. Br J Psychiatry 2011;199(1):5–7.

10. The Butterfly Foundation. Paying the price: the economic and social impact of eating disorders in Australia. 2012. Available at: http://thebutterflyfoundation. org.au/wp-content/uploads/2012/12/Butterfly_Report.pdf. Accessed November 9, 2015.

11. The Butterfly Foundation. Investing in need: cost-effective interventions for eating disorders. 2014. Available at: http://thebutterflyfoundation.org.au/wp-content/ uploads/2015/02/FULL-REPORT-Butterfly-Foundation-Investing-in-Need-cost-effective-interventions-for-eating-disorders-report.pdf.

12. Bratland-Sanda S, Sundgot-Borgen J. Eating disorders in athletes: overview of prevalence, risk factors and recommendations for prevention and treatment. Eur J Sport Sci 2013;13(5):499–508.

13. Carter JC, Stewart DA, Fairburn CG. Eating disorder examination questionnaire: norms for young adolescent girls. Behav Res Ther 2001;39(5):625–32.

14. Sangenis P, Drinkwater BL, Loucks A, et al. Position stand on the female athlete triad: IOC Medical Commission Working Group Women in sport. 2009;46. Available at: http://www.olympic.org/documents/reports/en/en_report_917.pdf. Accessed July 17, 2015.

15. Birch K. Female athlete triad. BMJ 2005;330(7485):244–6.

16. Zach KN, Smith Machin AL, Hoch AZ. Advances in management of the female athlete triad and eating disorders. Clin Sports Med 2011;30(3):551–73.

17. Tan J, Bloodworth A, McNamee M, et al. Investigating eating disorders in elite gymnasts: conceptual, ethical and methodological issues. Eur J Sport Sci 2012;14(1):1–9.

18. American Psychiatric Association. DSM-5. 2014. Available at: http://www.dsm5. org/Pages/Default.aspx.

19. World Health Organization. ICD-10. 2014. Available at: http://apps.who.int/ classifications/icd10/browse/2014/en#/.

20. Al-Adawi S, Bax B, Bryant-Waugh R, et al. Revision of ICD – status update on feeding and eating disorders. Adv Eat Disord 2013;1(1):10–20.

21. American Psychiatric Association. Feeding and eating disorders. In: Diagnostic and statistical manual of mental disorders. 5th edition (DSM-5). Arlington (VA): American Psychiatric Publishing; 2013. p. 1–2. http://dx.doi.org/10.1176/appi. books.9780890425596.323864.

22. Hudson JI, Hiripi E, Pope HG, et al. The prevalence and correlates of eating disorders in the National Comorbidity Survey Replication. Biol Psychiatry 2007;61(3): 348–58.

23. Fairburn CG, Cooper Z, Doll HA, et al. Risk factors for anorexia nervosa: three integrated case-control comparisons. Arch Gen Psychiatry 1995;56:468–76.

24. Janout V, Janoutová G. Eating disorders risk groups in the Czech Republic–cross-sectional epidemiologic pilot study. Biomed Pap Med Fac Univ Palacky Olomouc Czech Repub 2004;148(2):189–93.

25. Treasure JL, Wack ER, Roberts ME. Models as a high-risk group: the health implications of a size zero culture. Br J Psychiatry 2008;192(4):243–4.

26. Steinberg L, Silverberg SB. The vicissitudes of autonomy in early adolescence. Child Dev 2014;57(4):841–51.

27. Mond JM, Hay PJ, Rodgers B, et al. Eating Disorder Examination Questionnaire (EDE-Q): norms for young adult women. Behav Res Ther 2006;44(1):53–62.

28. Milos G, Spindler A, Schnyder U, et al. Instability of eating disorder diagnoses: prospective study. Br J Psychiatry 2005;187:573–8.

29. Reas DL, Øverås M, Rø O. Norms for the Eating Disorder Examination Questionnaire (EDE-Q) among high school and university men. Eat Disord 2012;20(5): 437–43.

30. Striegel-Moore RH, Bulik CM. Risk factors for eating disorders. Am Psychol 2007; 62(3):181–98.

31. Bulik CM, Sullivan PF, Kendler KS. An empirical study of the classification of eating disorders. Am J Psychiatry 2000;157(6):886–95.

32. Hope T, Tan J, Stewart A, et al. Anorexia nervosa and the language of authenticity. Hastings Cent Rep 2005;41(6):19–29.

33. Charland LC, Hope T, Stewart A, et al. Anorexia nervosa as a passion. Philos Psychiatr Psychol 2012;(4):353–65.

34. Beumont PJV. Compulsory treatment in anorexia nervosa. Br J Psychiatry 2000; 176:298.

35. Thiel A, Paul T. Compulsory treatment in anorexia nervosa. Psychother Psychosom Med Psychol 2014;57(3–4):128–35.

36. Roberts Strife S, Rickard K. The conceptualization of anorexia: the pro-ANA perspective. J Women Soc Work 2011;26(2):213–7.

37. Boughtwood D, Halse C. Other than obedient: girls' constructions of doctors and treatment regimes for anorexia nervosa. J Community Appl Soc Psychol 2010; 20(2):83–94.

38. Craigie J, Hope T, Tan J, et al. Agency, ambivalence and authenticity: the many ways in which anorexia nervosa can affect autonomy. Int J Law Context 2013;9(1):20–36. Available at: http://ezproxy.net.ucf.edu/login?url=http://search.ebscohost.com/login.aspx?direct=true&db=aph&AN=85634068&site=ehost-live.

39. Tan JOA, Stewart A, Fitzpatrick R, et al. Attitudes of patients with anorexia nervosa to compulsory treatment and coercion. Int J Law Psychiatry 2010;33(1): 13–9.

40. Kerr G, Dacyshyn A. The retirement experiences of elite, female gymnasts. J Appl Sport Psychol 2000;12(2):115–33.

41. Baxter-Jones ADG, Maffulli N. Intensive training in elite young female athletes. Br J Sports Med 2002;36(1):13–5.

42. McNamee M. Celebrating trust: virtues and rules in the ethical conduct of sports coaches. In: Mcnamee M, Parry SJ, editors. Ethics and sport. London: Routledge; 2002. p. 148–68.

43. Francisco R, Alarcão M, Narciso I. Aesthetic sports as high-risk contexts for eating disorders – young elite dancers and gymnasts perspectives. Span J Psychol 2012;15(1):265–74.

44. Nordin S, Harris G, Cumming J. Disturbed eating in young, competitive gymnasts: differences between three gymnastics disciplines. Eur J Sport Sci 2003; 3(5):1–14.

45. Garner DM, Garfinkel PE, Stancer HC, et al. Body image disturbances in anorexia nervosa and obesity. Psychosom Med 1976;38(5):327–36.

46. Fairburn CG, Beglin SJ. Assessment of eating disorder psychopathology: interview or self-report questionnaire? Int J Eat Disord 1994;16:363–70.

47. Beck A, Ward C, Mendelson M. Beck depression inventory. Arch Gen Psychiatry 1961;4(1995):561–71.

48. Rosenberg M. Society and the adolescent self-image. Princeton (NJ): Princeton University Press; 1965. Available at: http://www.bsos.umd.edu/socy/research/rosenberg.htm.

49. Mond JM, Hay PJ, Rodgers B, et al. Validity of the Eating Disorder Examination Questionnaire (EDE-Q) in screening for eating disorders in community samples. Behav Res Ther 2004;42(5):551–67.
50. Garner DM. Eating Attitudes Test (EAT-26): scoring and interpretation. 2004. Available at: http://www.eat-26.com/downloads.php.
51. Carter JC, Stewart DA, Fairburn CG. Eating disorder examination questionnaire: norms for young adolescent girls. Behav Res Ther 2001;39(5):625–32.
52. Mond JM, Hay PJ, Rodgers B, et al. Eating Disorder Examination Questionnaire (EDE-Q): norms for young adult women. Behav Res Ther 2006;44(1):53–62.
53. Wade TD, Byrne S, Bryant-Waugh R. The eating disorder examination: norms and construct validity with young and middle adolescent girls. Int J Eat Disord 2008; 41(6):551–8.
54. Luce KH, Crowther JH, Pole M. Eating Disorder Examination Questionnaire (EDE-Q): norms for undergraduate women. Int J Eat Disord 2008;41(3): 273–6.
55. Lavender JM, De Young KP, Anderson DA. Eating Disorder Examination Questionnaire (EDE-Q): norms for undergraduate men. Eat Behav 2010;11(2):119–21.
56. Bloodworth A, McNamee M, Tan J. Autonomy, eating disorders and elite sport. Sport Educ Soc, in press.
57. Bachner-Melman R, Zohar AH, Ebstein RP, et al. How anorexic-like are the symptom and personality profiles of aesthetic athletes? Med Sci Sports Exerc 2006; 38(4):628–36.
58. Krentz EM, Warschburger P. Sports-related correlates of disordered eating in aesthetic sports. Psychol Sport Exerc 2011;12(4):375–82.
59. Thompson RA, Sherman RT. 'Good athlete' traits and characteristics of anorexia nervosa: are they similar? Eat Disord 1999;7(3):181–90.
60. Mountjoy M, Sundgot-Borgen J, Burke L, et al. The IOC consensus statement: beyond the female athlete triad–Relative Energy Deficiency in Sport (RED-S). Br J Sports Med 2014;48(7):491–7.
61. Granger LR, Johnson CL, Malina RM, et al. National athletic trainers' association position statement: preventing, detecting, and managing disordered eating in athletes. J Athl Train 2008;43(1):80–108.
62. Sundgot-Borgen J, Meyer NL, Lohman TG, et al. How to minimise the health risks to athletes who compete in weight-sensitive sports review and position statement on behalf of the Ad Hoc Research Working Group on body composition, health and performance, under the auspices of the IOC medical commission. Br J Sports Med 2013;47(16):1012–22.
63. Laing EM, Massoni JA, Nickols-Richardson SM, et al. A prospective study of bone mass and body composition in female adolescent gymnasts. J Pediatr 2002;141(2):211–6.
64. Robinson TL, Snow-Harter C, Taaffe DR, et al. Gymnasts exhibit higher bone mass than runners despite similar prevalence of amenorrhea and oligomenorrhea. J Bone Miner Res 1995;10(1):26–35.
65. Burrows M, Shepherd H, Bird S, et al. The components of the female athlete triad do not identify all physically active females at risk. J Sports Sci 2007;25(12): 1289–97.
66. Vicente-Rodriguez G, Dorado C, Ara I, et al. Artistic versus rhythmic gymnastics: effects on bone and muscle mass in young girls. Int J Sports Med 2007;28(5): 386–93.
67. Hawton K, James A. Suicide and deliberate self harm in young people. BMJ 2005;330(7496):891–4.

68. Hawton K, Rodham K, Evans E, et al. Deliberate self harm in adolescents: self report survey in schools in England. BMJ 2002;325(7374):1207–11.

69. Kerr G, Berman E, De Souza MJ. Disordered eating in women's gymnastics: perspectives of athletes, coaches, parents, and judges. J Appl Sport Psychol 2006; 18(1):28–43.

70. Baxter-Jones ADG, Maffulli N, Mirwald RL. Does elite competition inhibit growth and delay maturation in some gymnasts? Probably not. Pediatr Exerc Sci 2003; 15(4):373–82.

71. O'Connor J, Lewis RD, Kirchner M, et al. Eating disorder symptoms in former female gymnasts: relations with body composition. Am J Clin Nutr 1996;64: 840–3.

72. Serpell L, Livingstone A, Neiderman M, et al. Anorexia nervosa: obsessive-compulsive disorder, obsessive-compulsive personality disorder, or neither? Clin Psychol Rev 2002;22(5):647–69.

73. Serpell L, Treasure J, Teasdale J, et al. Anorexia nervosa: friend or foe? Int J Eat Disord 1999;25:177–86.

74. Henderson J. Too thin to win. Athl Wkly 2012. Available at: http://www.athleticsweekly.com/0/admin/blog/too-thin-to-win/. Accessed July 17, 2015.

Ethics of Regulating Competition for Women with Hyperandrogenism

Silvia Camporesi, PhD, PhD

KEYWORDS

- Hyperandrogenism • Fairness • IAAF • Medicalization • Caster Semenya
- Dutee Chand

KEY POINTS

- IAAF Hyperandrogenism Regulations are flawed on a scientific level because it has not been proved that testosterone confers an advantage in competition.
- IAAF Hyperandrogenism Regulations raise issues of consistencies on two levels: other molecular and genetic variations that confer an advantage in competition are not considered unfair; and there is no upper limit for testosterone in the male category.
- IAAF Hyperandrogenism Regulations raise ethical issues at the level of implementation because the trigger for testing is visual perception and hence they pressure female athletes into conforming to stereotypical feminine standards.
- IAAF Hyperandrogenism Regulations raise medical concerns because they unnecessarily medicalize a condition (hyperandrogenism) in female athletes with long-term side effects.
- We need to be critical of the grounds on which the Court of Arbitration for Sport (CAS) has suspended the IAAF Hyperandrogenism Regulations on July 27, 2015, because CAS is buying into the IAAF flawed assumption that if there were a sufficient body of evidence to demonstrate a correlation between testosterone and competitive advantage, this would be unfair and would constitute grounds to reinstate the hyperandrogenism regulations.

INTRODUCTION

This article first briefly presents the case of Caster Semenya, which triggered the drafting of the International Association of Athletics Federations (IAAF; the international governing body regulating athletics competition worldwide) regulations on eligibility of female athletes with hyperandrogenism to compete in the female category. Then the IAAF regulations are critically analyzed from a scientific and ethical point of view. Finally the Court of Arbitration for Sport (CAS; international body that settles

Disclosure Statement: The author has no competing statements to disclose.
Department of Social Science, Health and Medicine, King's College London, D6, 2nd Floor, East Wing, London WC2R 2LS, UK
E-mail address: silvia.1.camporesi@kcl.ac.uk

sports disputes worldwide) landmark decision (July 2015) to suspend the regulations pending further evidence, and what this means for the future of sports, is discussed.

THE CASE OF CASTER SEMENYA

One cannot discuss the IAAF guidelines for regulating competition of women with hyperandrogenism without recalling the case of Caster Semenya, which prompted the guidelines. Caster Semenya competed at the Berlin IAAF Track Championship in 2009, where she won the 800 m with a time of 1:56.72, a total of 2.5 seconds ahead of the runner up. Only a few hours after the race the IAAF started an investigation into her gender. The IAAF reported that the "incredible improvement in the athlete's performance" triggered the investigation and compared her improvement with "the sort of dramatic breakthroughs that usually arouse suspicion of drug abuse."[1]

Complaints from Semenya's competitors not only to the large margin of her win, but also to her "butch appearance" were a trigger for investigation.[1] The IAAF banned Semenya from competitions during the investigation. Semenya was eventually reinstated to compete after an 11-month investigation but the results of her tests were never made public.

In 2009 there were no guidelines regulating gender testing, because the IAAF had abandoned all in 1991, as did the International Olympic Committee (IOC) in 1999.[2] As reported,[3] the IAAF argued that gender testing was no longer necessary because "modern sportswear was now so revealing that it seemed unfeasible that a man could masquerade as a woman,"[4(p7)] which had been the main concern underlying the gender testing regulations. After concerns for false-positive results at the Atlanta Olympic Games in 1996, in 1999 the IOC also removed the requirements for gender testing.

Semenya's case triggered the IAAF, in coordination with the IOC, to revisit the guidelines for when a woman should be allowed to compete as a woman. The new AAF Regulations Governing Eligibility of Females with Hyperandrogenism to Compete in Women's Competition came into force in May 2011, shortly followed by similar IOC policies.[4] Although neither the IAAF nor IOC mention explicitly a relationship between Caster Semenya and the regulations, this is apparent and an extensive body of critical literature has been written on the subject.[5]

THE INTERNATIONAL ASSOCIATION OF ATHLETICS FEDERATIONS REGULATIONS

Hyperandrogenism is the result of a set of naturally occurring conditions, such as polycystic ovary syndrome, where genetically female individuals produce higher levels of androgens. This condition may confer several phenotypic traits typically associated with masculinity, such as hirsutism and an increased muscle bulk.[6] Hyperandrogenism does not pose an immediate threat to the health of the person affected.

The IAAF and IOC policies require female athletes who do not fall within the limits of 100 ng/dL of testosterone to undergo androgen-suppressive therapy for up to 2 years to reduce the level of testosterone to compete as females. The unfair advantage thesis is the pervasive assumption underlying the construction of female categories in elite sports. Paragraph 6.5 of the IAAF policies on eligibility of women with hyperandrogenism to compete in women's competition states this quite clearly[3]:

The Expert Medical Panel shall recommend that the athlete is eligible to compete in women's competition if: (i) She has androgen levels below the normal male range; or (ii) She has androgen levels within the normal male range but has an androgen resistance such that she derives no competitive advantage from having androgen levels in the normal male range.

The burden of proof to demonstrate that female athletes with hyperandrogenism do not derive a competitive advantage from the excess testosterone is on the athlete. The assumption of the IAAF regulations is that hyperandrogenism provides an unfair advantage and disrupts the level playing field, and that the pharmacologic treatment required to reduce the testosterone level is a means to ensure the level playing field in competition.

The regulations have been widely criticized. I among others have coauthored papers arguing that the IAAF Regulations are unfair on many different levels and should be withdrawn.[1,7–12] In what follows I outline the main lines of critique relative to the unfairness of the IAAF Regulations in terms of absence of conclusive evidence, of internal and external inconsistencies, of visual perception as a trigger for testing, and of unnecessary medicalization.

TESTOSTERONE CONFERS A COMPETITIVE ADVANTAGE: CASE NOT PROVED

As read in the regulation: "The difference in athletic performance between males and females is known to be predominantly due to higher levels of androgenic hormones in males resulting in increased strength and muscle development."[3(p1)] The authors of the IAAF Regulations also write that "In events where androgenization provides a powerful advantage, women want to compete against alike, not against women with a degree of hyperandrogenism that gives them a male physiology."[13(p65)]

But Is The Case Proved?

As reviewed by Karkazis and Jordan-Young,[14] there are many unknowns regarding how testosterone works with regard to athleticism, but what is clear is that testosterone cannot be used to predict who is going to perform better, nor can it be used to infer that people who perform better have more testosterone. Moreover, although the reference range for testosterone for men is between 300 and 1200 ng/dL and for women it does not exceed, on average, 100 ng/dL, it has been observed that testosterone concentrations vary according to several factors, such as exposure to exogenous hormones (eg, estrogen and thyroxine), the time of the day, and the age of the individual.[15] Evidence has also been provided against the supposed correlation between high levels of endogenous testosterone and an advantage in competition from athletes with nonfunctioning testosterone.[16]

That the correlation between levels of testosterone and competitive advantage has not been proved is the argument that led on July 27, 2015 to the suspension of the regulations by the CAS. But even if this correlation could be unequivocally proved, I argue that this would not constitute and unfair advantage. Reasons to reinstate the regulations are discussed next.

INCONSISTENCIES IN THE REGULATIONS

Singling out, and setting a limit on, hyperandrogenism from other biologic variations that may confer a genetic advantage is an inconsistent policy: there are plenty of other genetic variations that are not regulated by the IAAF and, even though advantageous for athletic performance, they are not considered unfair for competition.

More than 200 genetic variations have been identified that provide an advantage in elite sport, which affect a variety of functions including blood flow to muscles, muscle structure, oxygen transport, lactate turnover, and energy production. Endurance athletes in particular have been shown to have mitochondrial variations that increase aerobic capacity and endurance.[17] An increasing number of performance-enhancing polymorphisms are identified by sports geneticists.[18] For example, elite sprinters have a higher frequency of a polymorphism at the level of the gene coding for actinin-3 protein, a component of the contractile apparatus in fast skeletal muscle fibers, which plays a pivotal role in generating contractile force in sprints.[17] Mutations at the level of the myostatin gene that confer an increased muscle bulk have been identified.[19]

A volume commissioned by the IOC Medical Commission titled *Genetic and Molecular Aspects of Sport Performance* was recently published.[20] Athletes with naturally occurring, endogenous genetic or biologic variations are celebrated as a source of inborn excellence, and children born with such mutations are encouraged to pursue a career in sport. It seems ironic that at the same time that the IOC commissions research on the genetic variations of sport performance, it does not see the inconsistencies inherent in the IAAF and IOC policies on hyperandrogenism.

Indeed, elite athletes derive advantages from a range of endogenous biologic variations, and hyperandrogenism is only one of these variations. As pointed out by Sullivan[21]: "The fact is the playing field [in elite sports] has never been level. There will always be genetic variations that provide a competitive edge for some athletes over others. We readily accept the genetic, athletic gifts that elite athletes possess without trying to find ways to "level the playing field."

In addition, the IAAF and IOC policies raise concerns in terms of internal consistency. Indeed, if we buy into the IAAF assumption that higher levels of testosterones confer an unfair advantage in competition and that it is necessary to set an upper limit to redress the level playing field, then one wonders why there is not an upper limit for the male category. On the contrary, as pointed out by Sonksen and coworkers[16(p1)]: "For many years now, natural advantage among male athletes has not been policed and reduced in sports, but on the contrary has been admired and celebrated." The IAAF/IOC regulations not only raise issues of consistency, but are also unfair at the level of implementation, as discussed next.

VISUAL PERCEPTION AS A TRIGGER FOR TESTING AND THE BURDEN TO PERFORM FEMININITY

Visual perception functions as the visual trigger for testing. The Tanner-Whitehouse Scoring sheet used by the IAAF as one of nine "clinical signs" used to identify possible hyperandrogenism in female athletes.[22]

Although the IAAF no longer uses the term "femininity" in its regulations, they nonetheless display a marked focus on what are broadly considered to be feminine physical characteristics, such as (lack of) body hair and the size and shape of breasts.[22] Hence, female athletes who do not conform to "normal" social standards of femininity are the targets for testing. Hence, there is an increasing pressure on women athletes to "perform heteronormative standards femininity" to avoid having their gender called into question.[8] In addition, as argued by Teetzel[23(p20)]

Subjecting women athletes who look more muscular, androgynous, or masculine than their competitors to sex verification procedures, and requiring them to plead their cases to a panel of experts to continue competing in the women's category, [...] is also reminiscent of witch hunts, and has the potential to be applied in racist and classist ways.

It is worth noting that so far all the women who have been targeted by the IAAF guidelines are women from developing countries, as reported by Macur.[24] The standard stereotype of femininity to which athletes are pressured to conform is white, and "flawless." Hence one can see in these policies the intersection of different narratives of gender, race, and medical imperialism.[5] This supports the claim that female athletes who do not conform to heteronormative standards of femininity are targets of the testing, as was the case for Caster Semenya.

UNNECESSARY MEDICALIZATION

Hyperandrogenism does not pose an immediate threat to the health of the person affected. Medical evidence shows that high level of androgens only increase the risk of hirsutism, acne, and possibly alopecia, and have other virilizing cutaneous manifestations,[6] but none of these augmented risks is incompatible with physical activity or participation in elite sport. There are many women who are not athletes affected by hyperandrogenism (between 10% and 15% of women are affected by polycystic ovary syndrome[6]), but they do not have to take androgen suppressive therapy or undergo surgeries, including feminizing plastic surgeries that are recommended by the regulations and that have nothing to do with levels of testosterone.

From 2011 to 2015 several cases have been prompted by the regulations. As reported by Fénichel and coauthors,[25] four unnamed female athletes were found to have levels of testosterone higher than 10 nmol/L. The article does not report where the athletes are from but states that they came "from rural or mountainous regions of developing countries."[25(pE1057)] The athletes were referred to the Reproductive Endocrinology Department at the Nice and Montpellier University Hospitals in France, which collaborates with sports governing bodies.

The four athletes were all subjected to unnecessary medicalization procedures that had nothing to do with reducing testosterone levels in sport: a "partial clitoridectomy with a bilateral gonadectomy, followed by a deferred feminizing vaginoplasty and estrogen replacement therapy."[25] The article also reports that sports authorities then allowed them to continue competing in the female category 1 year after gonadectomy.[25]

As noted by Sonksen and coworkers,[16(p2)] the additional feminizing procedures described by Fenichel and colleagues[25] are "particularly alarming" and the notion that the policies emanate out of a concern for the health of the athletes[13] needs to be contested. The choice of treatment for the four athletes is inconsistent with clinical practice, whereby outside the field of play women with hyperandrogenism are not required to undergo clitoridectomies or androgen-suppressive therapies, which raise health sequelae in the near and long term.[16] Hence, surgical and medical procedures are unnecessary from a clinical practice point of view, but are only necessary as a condition to re-enter the field of play. In this respect, the rationale for imposing treatment lies outside of considerations of beneficence cheered in medical ethics.[13]

The most recent and famous case, which has led to the appeal to the CAS, that of Dutee Chand, is discussed later.

BURDEN OF PROOF AND OF COST ON ATHLETES

The burden of proof to demonstrate androgen resistance (and hence, not to derive an "advantage" from higher levels of testosterone) falls on the athletes[3]:

> The burden of proof shall be on the athlete to establish, where applicable, that she has an androgen resistance such that she derives no competitive advantage from androgen levels in the normal male range and the standard of proof in such a case shall be by a balance of probabilities (paragraph 6.6 of the rules).

Not only is the burden of proof on the athlete, but so is the burden of cost for the treatment. Indeed, although the policies provide explicit recommendation of treatment, they also explicitly state that they do not cover the costs for medical intervention[3]:

> The athlete shall be responsible for complying with her prescribed medical treatment during the period of Return to Competition Monitoring and shall provide the IAAF Medical Department with satisfactory evidence of such compliance, as it may request (paragraph 7.4 of the IAAF 2011 regulations).

Such costs rest on the shoulders of the athletes or their families. As noted by Slater,[26] many of these athletes come from humble social backgrounds and through their participation in world track events are not only providing for themselves but also for their families. When the policies target them, not only are the athletes deprived of the opportunity to compete, but also of the means to make a living for them and for their families. It does not seem an exaggeration to say that the burden for the athlete, which we have seen is physical, psychological, and economical in nature, disproportionately affects individuals from developing countries who already find themselves embedded into complex patterns of systematic disadvantage.

DUTEE CHAND'S APPEAL TO COURT OF ARBITRATION FOR SPORT AND THE SUSPENSION OF REGULATIONS

Dutee Chand, a promising 19-year-old Indian sprinter (in 2012 she became a national champion in the under-18 category in the 100 m event), was disqualified just days before the beginning of the Commonwealth Games in Glasgow in July 2014 after a medical test determined that her levels of testosterone were higher than the 10 nmol/L limit set by the IAAF.[26] According to IAAF regulations, if Chand were able to reduce her androgen levels she would be allowed to resume competition. Chand refused to do so and has appealed to the CAS, with financial support from the sports ministry of India.[27] The appeal of Dutee Chand took place at CAS headquarters in Lausanne, Switzerland, March 26 to 28, 2015.[27]

On July 27, 2015, the CAS announced that the regulations on hyperandrogenism have been suspended for the next 2 years to give the IAAF the opportunity to provide the CAS with scientific evidence about the quantitative relationship between enhanced testosterone levels and improved athletic performance in hyperandrogenic athletes. If the IAAF is unable to produce such evidence, the regulations will be considered void.[28]

The suspension allows Dutee Chand to now resume competition. The decision obviously clears the ground not only for her but also for other female athletes with hyperandrogenism. But a closer look at the CAS Interim Award gives reason to worry.

Indeed, the CAS panel has concluded that there is "presently insufficient evidence about the degree of advantage that androgen-sensitive hyperandrogenic females enjoy over non-hyperandrogenic females" (paragraph 522, Interim Award CAS),[29] and has asked IAAF to demonstrate a "correlation" between levels of testosterone in female athletes and competitive advantage. CAS has requested to prove that there is indeed an advantage derived by higher levels of testosterone. Although the suspension of the regulations is clearly reason to rejoice in the short term for Dutee Chand, it is concerning that the proviso for the suspension of the regulations falls within the scientific track of the IAAF. The CAS panel explicitly states that the IAAF assumption (that increased testosterone confers an advantage) "may well be proved valid" (paragraph 543, Interim Award)[29] but sufficient evidence has not yet been provided to show evidence of correlation, and currently the "onus of proof remains" on the IAAF (paragraph 534, Interim Award).[29] The CAS is buying into the assumption that if it were proved that testosterone provided an athletic advantage, then the regulations should be reinstated.

To the contrary, as I have described here, and have argued for more extensively elsewhere,[30] even if testosterone did confer an athletic advantage that could be proved by the IAAF on submission of further evidence, this advantage would not be unfair and would not constitute grounds for the reinstatement of the regulations.

SUMMARY

This article shows that the IAAF Regulations are problematic on many levels, from a scientific and from an ethical point of view. The medicalized discourse the IAAF and IOC require runs counter to the very same principle of fair play that the policies purport to protect. As noted by Sonksen and coworkers,[16(p2)] "one of the 'fundamental principles' of fairness in sport is nondiscrimination, namely that opportunities to participate and compete be open to all, regardless of economic, social, religious, racial/ethnic, and linguistic background or sexual orientation, as evidenced in Principle 6 of the Olympic Charter."

Although the CAS decision clears the track for competition by Dutee Chand and by other female athletes with hyperandrogenism, we should not consider this a happy ending because of the grounds on which the suspension of the regulations has been granted. Indeed, the IAAF has noted that it will work toward producing the evidence needed to reinstate the regulations.[31] We should be critical of the proviso the suspension has been granted on by the CAS, and prepare to fight for women's rights to compete based on fairness and without unnecessary medicalization.

REFERENCES

1. Camporesi S, Maugeri P. Caster Semenya: sport, categories and the creative role of ethics. J Med Ethics 2010;36(6):378–9.
2. Elsas LJ, Ljungqvist A, Ferguson-Smith MA, et al. Gender verification of female athletes. Genet Med 2000;2(4):249–54.
3. International Association for Athletics Federations Hyperandrogenism Regulation. Available at: http://www.iaaf.org/about-iaaf/documents/medical. Accessed August 1, 2015.
4. Heggie V. Testing sex and gender in sports; reinventing, reimagining and reconstructing histories. Endeavour 2010;34(4):157–63.
5. Olivesi A, Montanola S, editors. Gender sport, and ethics: the case of Caster Semenya. London: Routledge; 2016. Ethics in Sport Series.
6. Housman E, Reynolds RV. Polycystic ovary syndrome: a review for dermatologists: part I. Diagnosis and manifestations. J Am Acad Dermatol 2014;71(5): 847.e1–10.
7. Karkazis K, Jordan-Young R, Davis G, et al. Out of bounds? A critique of the new policies on hyperandrogenism in elite female athletes. Am J Bioeth 2012;12(7): 3–16.
8. Camporesi S. The burden of proving femininity in athletics. Why Dutee Chand should be allowed to compete. Huff Post Women March 25th, 2015. Available at: http://www.huffingtonpost.com/silvia-camporesi/the-burden-of-proving-femininity-in-athletics_b_6940562.html. Accessed August 1, 2015.
9. Camporesi S. Clear Skies overhead for Dutee Chand, but clouds loom on the horizon. Huff post sports July 30th, 2015. Available at: http://www.huffingtonpost.com/

silvia-camporesi/clear-skies-overhead-for-_b_7896924.html. Accessed August 1, 2015.

10. Behrensen M. In the halfway house of ill repute: gender verification under a different name, still no contribution to fair play. Sport Ethics Philos 2013;7(4): 450–66.

11. Cooky C, Dworkin SL. Policing the boundaries of sex: a critical examination of gender verification and the Caster Semenya controversy. J Sex Res 2013; 50(2):103–11.

12. Davis P, Edwards L. The new IOC and IAAF policies on female eligibility: old emperor, new clothes? Sport Ethics Philos 2014;8(1):44–56.

13. Bermon S, Ritzén M, Hirschberg AL, et al. Are the new policies on hyperandrogenism in elite female athletes really out of bounds? Response to "Out of bounds? A critique of the new policies on hyperandrogenism in elite female athletes. Am J Bioeth 2013;13(5):63–5.

14. Karkazis K, Jordan-Young R. The Harrison Bergeron olympics. Am J Bioeth 2013; 13(5):66–9.

15. Bostwick JM, Joyner MJ. The limits of acceptable biological variation in elite athletes: should sex ambiguity be treated differently from other advantageous genetic traits? Mayo Clin Proc 2012;87(6):508.

16. Sonksen P, Ferguson-Smith MA, Bavington LD, et al. Medical and ethical concerns regarding women with hyperandrogenism and elite sport. J Clin Endocrinol Metab 2015;100(3):825–7.

17. Ostrander EA, Huson HJ, Ostrander GK. Genetics of athletic performance. Annu Rev Genomics Hum Genet 2009;10:407–29.

18. Pitsiladis Y, Wang G, Wolfarth B, et al. Genomics of elite sporting performance: what little we know and necessary advances. Br J Sports Med 2013;47(9): 550–5.

19. Lee SJ. Sprinting without myostatin: a genetic determinant of athletic prowess. Trends Genet 2007;23(10):475–7.

20. Bouchard C, Hoffman EP, editors. The encyclopaedia of sports medicine: an IOC medical commission publication, genetic and molecular aspects of sports performance, vol. 18. John Wiley & Sons; 2011.

21. Sullivan CF. Gender verification and gender policies in elite sport eligibility and "fair play". Journal of Sport and Social Issues 2011;35(4):400–19.

22. IAAF Hyperandrogenism Regulations – Appendices C. Available at: http://www.iaaf.org/about-iaaf/documents/medical. Accessed August 1, 2015.

23. Teetzel S. The onus of inclusivity: sport policies and the enforcement of the women's category in sport. J Philos Sport 2014;41(1):113–27.

24. Macur J. Fighting for the body she was born with. New York Times 2014. Available at: http://www.nytimes.com/2014/10/07/sports/sprinter-dutee-chand-fights-ban-over-her-testosterone-level.html?_r=0. Accessed August 1, 2015.

25. Fénichel P, Paris F, Philibert P, et al. Molecular diagnosis of 5α-reductase deficiency in 4 elite young female athletes through hormonal screening for hyperandrogenism. J Clin Endocrinol Metab 2013;98(6):E1055–9.

26. Molloy PM. Indian athlete Dutee Chand disqualified after failing so-called gender test bustle July 24th, 2014. Available at: http://www.bustle.com/articles/33066-indian-sprinter-dutee-chand-disqualified-after-failing-a-so-called-gender-test. Accessed August 1, 2015.

27. Dutee Chand: Indian sprinter starts appeal against hormone ban test BBC Sports March 23rd, 2015. Available at: http://www.bbc.com/sport/0/athletics/32015227. Accessed August 1, 2015.

28. Court of arbitration of sport press release on suspension of hyperandrogenism regulations July 27th, 2015. Available at: http://www.tas-cas.org/fileadmin/user_upload/Media_Release_3759_FINAL.pdf. Accessed August 1, 2015.

29. Court of arbitration of sport interim award on suspension of hyperandrogenism regulations July 27th, 2015. Available at: http://www.tas-cas.org/fileadmin/user_upload/award_internet.pdf. Accessed August 1, 2015.

30. Camporesi S, Maugeri P. Unfair advantage and the myth of the level playing field in IAAF and IOC policies on hyperandrogenism: when is it fair to be a woman?. In: Olivesi A, Montanola S, editors. Gender sport, and ethics: the case of Caster Semenya. London: Routledge; 2016. Ethics in Sport Series.

31. IAAF Press Release commenting on Interim Award issued by the CAS on IAAF's Hyperandrogenism regulations July 27th, 2015. Available at: http://www.iaaf.org/news/press-release/hyperandrogenism-regulations-cas-dutee-chand. Accessed August 1, 2015.

The Ethics of Sports Medicine Research

Robert J. Stewart, MD*, Bruce Reider, MD

KEYWORDS

- Research ethics • Sports medicine ethics • Declaration of Helsinki
- Ethical guidelines for research • Ethical controversies in research

KEY POINTS

- Significant changes have taken place over the past century regarding research ethics, allowing the establishment of numerous codes and guidelines.
- As pioneering treatment options are developed, reliance on evidence-based medicine is critical.
- Treating surgeons rely on research data that have been compiled and disseminated in an ethical and honest manner. This serves to avoid compromising patient care.
- The necessity for conducting ethical research is paramount, and use of the Declaration of Helsinki guidelines is essential for a safe and informed sports medicine practice.

RESEARCH ETHICS: BACKGROUND

Events of the late nineteenth century and surrounding World War II spawned concerns about how research was conducted, which led to the foundations of modern research ethics. In the late nineteenth century, yellow fever was a raging epidemic in Cuba. Giuseppe Sanarelli, an Italian bacteriologist, injected 5 people with an organism that he thought caused yellow fever, resulting in severe harm and wide criticism.[1,2] After this incident, the US Surgeon General commissioned Walter Reed to identify the cause of yellow fever. Reed developed ethical guidelines for this research, which were implemented by the US Army's Yellow Fever Board. This Board is considered the predecessor of today's Research Ethics Committee (REC).[1]

Later, the Nuremberg Code of 1947 was drafted in connection with the Nuremberg trials after World War II. The main principles of the Code were that informed consent is necessary, that research should yield results that are for the good of society, and that

Disclosure: The authors have nothing to disclose.
Department of Orthopaedics and Rehabilitation Medicine, The University of Chicago Medicine, 5841 South Maryland Avenue, MC3079, Chicago, IL 60614, USA
* Corresponding author.
E-mail address: robert.stewart@uchospitals.edu

Clin Sports Med 35 (2016) 303–314
http://dx.doi.org/10.1016/j.csm.2015.10.009
0278-5919/16/$ – see front matter © 2016 Elsevier Inc. All rights reserved.

risks to research subjects be minimized.[3-5] Since the Nuremberg Code, other principles and codes have been established to foster ethical research, including the following:

- The Declaration of Helsinki (1964)
- The Belmont Report (1979)
- International Council for Harmonisation (ICH) Good Clinical Practices (GCP)
- International Standards Organization 14155
- Code of Federal Regulations

The Declaration of Helsinki (DoH), adopted in 1964 by the World Medical Association (WMA), is a statement of ethical principles for medical research involving human subjects.[6] This document is the subject of much discussion in this article.

In 1974, the National Commission for the Protection of Human Subjects of Biomedical and Behavior Research began to formulate basic ethical principles as the foundation of conducting research involving human subjects.[7] Published in 1979, The Belmont Report became this foundation, emphasizing the following basic ethical principles:

- Respect for persons
- Beneficence
- Justice

Respect for persons involves obtaining informed consent and treating subjects autonomously. Importantly, it also pertains to protecting those with less autonomy; for example, an individual incapable of self-determination. Beneficence can be thought of as 2 general concepts: do no harm and maximize possible benefits while minimizing possible harms.[7] Justice refers to the question of who ought to receive the benefits of research and bear its burdens. An example of injustice was the Tuskegee syphilis study in the 1940s, which exploited disadvantaged, rural black men to study the natural course of syphilis. These subjects were never given the option to quit the study to receive adequate treatment, even when penicillin became available as the drug of choice to treat syphilis in 1947. Astonishingly, this study continued for 40 years from the time the first subject was enrolled in 1932.[8]

The ICH was founded in 1990 and brings together drug regulatory authorities and the pharmaceutical industries of Europe, Japan, and the United States. Its GCP guidelines were finalized in 1996 and implemented by the European Union and the US Food and Drug Administration (FDA).[9] The International Organization for Standardization (ISO) is an independent, nongovernmental organization with 163 member countries that provides specifications to ensure quality. ISO 14155 was most recently amended in 2011 and addresses GCP for the design, conduct, recording, and reporting of clinical investigations of medical devices for human subjects.[10] The final guideline for conducting ethical research is the Code of Federal Regulations. In 1991, the Federal Policy for the Protection of Human Subjects, or Common Rule, was published. All of these regulations were developed with The Belmont Report as the foundation.[11]

DECLARATION OF HELSINKI: BACKGROUND

Without diminishing the value of the principles and codes described earlier, the DoH and how it relates to orthopedic sports medicine is discussed here. It is important to emphasize that the DoH was born from an association of physicians, the WMA. Hence, it is primarily directed at physicians who face a unique dilemma when conducting research on human subjects. They have the responsibility to investigate the safety and efficacy of interventions on human subjects in an attempt to advance treatment options. However, at times this can seem to conflict with their fundamental obligation to do no harm. The DoH was the first international regulation to address this dilemma.[12]

Although the DoH is recognized as the most cited document on international research ethics,[13] it has both proponents and naysayers[14–16]; its contents are decided via the democratic method of voting, so there are always aspects of the document that require compromise or indetermination.[15]

The DoH has been described as the North Star[17] and the gold standard[18] of medical research ethics.[15] The document has been through 7 revisions and more than doubled in length. Many consider it a living document that continually adapts to changing ethical challenges. This property has allowed it to remain relevant over a long period of time.[12,19] The fluidity of the document is a priority of the WMA to meet current and future challenges in response to developments in medical research.[20] Sports medicine evolves quickly and requires fluidity to practice. Because of this, it makes sense that a document such as the DoH is particularly relevant to this field. The DoH has been organized into 12 titled sections containing 37 numbered bullet points. Throughout the remainder of this article, each paragraph is referred to by its number.

DECLARATION OF HELSINKI: APPLICATION OF PRINCIPLES

In paragraph 2, the preamble of the DoH states that, in accordance with the mandate of the WMA, the document primarily addresses physicians. In reality, its guidelines are for all health care providers involved in clinical research. The intended audience (physicians) of this document is apparent when considering paragraph 3, which recalls an overriding obligation of physicians from the Declaration of Geneva of the WMA: "The health of my patient will be my first consideration." Orthopedic surgeons must constantly remind themselves of the inherent vulnerability of their patients, and their promise to do no harm.[12]

Paragraph 5 introduces the physician's dilemma to protect the welfare of individual patients in addition to the welfare of humanity. It states that medical progress is based on research that ultimately must include studies involving human subjects. Various ethical code documents address this dilemma in different ways. For instance, the ICH-GCP seems to protect the research and welfare of humanity more than the individual in the research, because of its emphasis on the efficacy of drugs involved in trials involving human subjects.[16] In contrast, in paragraph 8, the DoH places emphasis on protecting the welfare of the individual: "While the primary purpose of medical research is to generate new knowledge, this goal can never take precedence over the rights and interests of individual research subjects." Sham surgery has been a recent topic of ethical discussion involving orthopedic sports medicine. It exemplifies the quandary that physicians face in trying to maximize benefit to humanity without compromising the well-being of individuals. It has been argued that sham surgery is unethical because it fails to minimize risk the same way a placebo-controlled drug trial does.[21] Regardless of a physician's belief regarding sham surgery, the patient's welfare should take precedence.

Paragraph 6, some of which is new from the 2000 revision, seems to favor research and the welfare of humanity more than the welfare of the individual being researched. However, as paragraph 1 states, "The declaration is intended to be read as a whole and each of its constituent paragraphs should be applied with consideration of all other relevant paragraphs," so the individual being researched has been protected elsewhere in the document and should not be forgotten. Paragraph 6 challenges physicians to continue research on already established treatments, stating that "Even the best proven interventions must be evaluated continually through research for their safety, effectiveness, efficiency, accessibility and quality." This statement could elicit much controversy regarding the ethical tension[22] between protecting research subjects and the necessary "freedom of research to facilitate scientific progress as a public good."[23] It is easy for orthopedic surgeons to relate to the desire to challenge the "best proven interventions" when considering treatment options of their own patients.

Another change made in the 2000 revision of the DoH was to paragraph 10. This paragraph broaches the subject of relating law and ethics, which is a complex issue. Before 2000, the DoH seemed to act as guidelines that did not supersede national regulations. The document now acts as a minimum set of international standards to which physicians around the world should aspire.[22] This set of standards should not be compromised or eliminated for a national or international ethical, legal, or regulatory requirement. This issue of relating law and ethics is important in sports medicine research involving adult stem cells.[24] For example, a recent study involving knee injections of allogeneic mesenchymal stem cells after knee arthroscopy required additional regulatory guidance from the FDA.[25]

Orthopedic surgery involves treating a diverse group of patients. Racial and ethnic differences have been shown to affect outcomes in orthopedic patients.[26] It is critical to have results from research studies that can be generalized so physicians can make sound evidence-based treatment decisions. Paragraph 13 addresses populations that are underrepresented in research by demanding they have appropriate access to participation in research. This demand is important not only for the affected populations but also because it emphasizes the need to perform research on populations that are likely to be within the exclusion criteria. These criteria include pregnant or lactating women, children, and the elderly,[27] none of whom are immune to sports-related injuries. In terms of ethnic underrepresentation, historical issues of recruitment and retention of African American populations into clinical trials comes to the fore. Past unethical experimentation has reinforced African American and other minorities' doubts about the medical system, which has led to a decreased likelihood of enrolling, or completing, a research study.[28]

In paragraphs 16, 17, and 18, the DoH addresses the complex issue of weighing risk and burdens on subjects versus the potential benefits of the research. RECs have the serious responsibility of identifying and weighing the risks and benefits.[29] On an institutional level, an REC is typically known as an institutional review board (IRB). Some of the REC's most important functions are described in these paragraphs of the DoH, which state that the potential benefits must outweigh the risks (paragraph 16), measures must be taken to minimize the risks (paragraph 17), and "when the risks are found to outweigh the potential benefits or when there is conclusive proof of definitive outcomes" (paragraph 18) the study should be assessed to continue, modify, or stop.

Orthopedic surgeons encounter instances of calculating risk versus benefit on a daily basis when treating patients. Conducting research is not exempt from this process and is an exercise in risk management. The main reason for initiating research is because of clinicians' persistent dubiety regarding risks and benefits of the treatments provided to patients.[30] The previous discussion of placebo (sham) surgery trials is an example of this topic.

A recent sham surgery trial[31] involving arthroscopic partial meniscectomy is controversial, given that some clinicians think that simply entering a joint with instruments and saline may have confounding effects.[32] Another contentious aspect of the study is whether it is ethically sound in terms of risks and benefits. Some clinicians have argued that, although performing sham knee surgery is controversial, evaluating the treatment effectiveness of degenerative knee disorders demands clear answers and the potential benefits of the study design outweigh the risks.[32] Others think that this type of study is not ethical and have stated their reasons to ignore it.[33] There is no doubt that the placebo surgical trial concept is fraught with ethical controversy, most of which involves weighing risk to the patient versus the potential benefit of the findings.

RECs are discussed in paragraph 23 of the DoH. This paragraph is one of the most important in the document, which is possibly why it was given its own section. Although it has been argued that the DoH is too ambiguous, this section is explicit in stating that the REC approval process is not optional. Some other salient features of the review process are clearly described[15]:

- The review process must be performed before the study begins.
- The committee must be transparent, independent, and qualified.
- The committee must know the local and international laws and regulations of the places where the research is taking place, but these must not detract from the protections that the DoH offers the research subjects.
- The committee must perform ongoing monitoring of the investigation.
- The investigator must submit a summary report to the committee when the study is complete, indicating the findings and conclusions.

Ethics committees must operate within the confines of local laws and regulations, and in accordance with the DoH. This facet of RECs (or IRBs) makes them a critical component of ethical research. It provides investigators with ethical guidelines but also has the flexibility to adapt these guidelines to local norms. By providing independent ethics committees with this right, the DoH recognizes the diverse environments in which research is conducted and the need to adapt the basic principles of research ethics within each research proposal. When evaluating the current status of ethics committee review and approval in the medical literature, several reviews have shown that some disciplines have poor documentation.[34–36] One group found a 22% rate of reporting ethics committee approval in a particular orthopedics journal.[37] Publisher policy varies when it comes to investigators providing documentation of ethical review for submitted research.

When dealing with diverse research environments, the concept of vulnerable groups and individuals must be understood. Paragraphs 19 and 20 introduce the subject of research on groups or individuals considered to be vulnerable. This section of the DoH has been revised in the most recent 2013 version, emphasizing special protection for vulnerable subjects because of their "increased likelihood of being wronged or of incurring additional harm." Some people argue that this section specifically addresses the poor and disadvantaged. For this reason, the group is vulnerable because they have limited access to care, not because they are at increased risk of being harmed.[38] Regardless of what group or individual is shown as vulnerable, certain individuals remain more prone than others to exploitation in research. In addition to the disadvantaged, medical students and employees, armed service members, student athletes, and children are all vulnerable in sports medicine research. Clinicians must always be mindful of this and conduct research with the knowledge that certain people may feel obligated to participate, even if they would rather not.[15]

Transitioning from the individuals who are being used for research, the section titled "Scientific Requirements and Research Protocols" addresses some important concepts that focus on specific responsibilities of the researcher. Paragraph 21 states that medical research must "be based on a thorough knowledge of the scientific literature" and "other relevant sources of information." By including this statement, the

DoH is saying that research conducted without sufficient knowledge of the current state of the topic investigated is unethical.[15] Paragraph 22 specifies that for a study to be ethically sound it must have a research protocol that includes "a statement of the ethical considerations involved … [and] information regarding funding, sponsors, institutional affiliations, potential conflicts of interest, incentives for subjects and information regarding provisions for treating and/or compensating subjects." This information is not trivial and, when considered together, it becomes obvious that the DoH is trying to encourage well-designed research that benefits the medical community. The importance of this section cannot be overemphasized. To uphold the integrity of orthopedic research, bad research needs to be vetted during the publication process. Going forward, it helps to remember that poor-quality research leads to increased risk to patients and may preclude any benefits from treatments. It cannot be denied that orthopedic sports medicine literature has published results from weak studies. However, a recently published review article concluded that there is an increasing proportion of prospective, comparative studies in sports medicine.[15,39]

The last sentence in paragraph 22 has raised significant debate. It states that, "… the protocol must also describe appropriate arrangements for post-trial provisions." In the 2008 version of the DoH the term "provisions" was difficult to interpret and various authorities have made comments criticizing the DoH for its presence.[12,40] In the 2013 revision of the DoH, paragraph 34 was written to elaborate on what provisions mean: "In advance of a clinical trial, sponsors, researchers, and host country governments should make provisions for post-trial access for all participants who still need an intervention identified as beneficial in the trial." This elaboration runs the risk of deterring some research from occurring because of concern of a costly obligation to treat participants after the research is complete.[16,41] The practicality of providing access to "an intervention identified as beneficial in the trial" has been called into question because of the elapsed time between the end of a study and getting an intervention approved for use by regulatory authorities. Furthermore, an intervention normally requires additional studies to prove its efficacy. Although the DoH provided a further description of posttrial provisions with the inclusion of paragraph 34, it does not explain how sponsors, researchers, and governments would share the expense of providing continued care.[42]

The vagueness of the statements involving posttrial provisions has been most contentious in its relation to chronic medical conditions. However, it can easily be translated to discussions in orthopedic sports medicine. For instance, an investigator evaluating the effectiveness of different injection therapies for posttraumatic arthrosis may be deterred from this research by the fear of facing increased time and expense based on the posttrial provision statements. If taken in the context of surgical interventions, a literal interpretation of this portion of the DoH could have daunting implications for researchers. For example, if a single study compares 2 different surgical interventions and one of them clearly has a better outcome, does this mean that patients who underwent the surgery with a worse outcome are entitled to the surgery shown to be superior[15]?

Paragraph 24 of the DoH is much less controversial and is under the section "Privacy and Confidentiality." The document states that, "Every precaution must be taken to protect the privacy of research subjects and the confidentiality of their personal information." Within the United States, the Health Insurance Portability and Accountability Act (HIPPA) Privacy Rule took effect in 2003. Its purpose is to protect the privacy of the health information of individuals. Some investigators think that the Privacy Rule has hindered research, particularly the ability to perform retrospective, chart reviews or prospective studies that involve contacting patients for follow-up information.[43] One study noted that the proportion of follow-up surveys completed decreased from 96% to 34% after the HIPPA Privacy Rule was implemented.[44] Orthopedic sports medicine research includes many retrospective chart reviews and prospective studies involving patient-reported outcome surveys. This specialty is affected by these regulations, but the importance of privacy and confidentiality of the human subjects cannot be overemphasized. With the advent of electronic medical records, more changes have taken place regarding laws and regulations to protect patient privacy. Research has not been isolated from the effects of this regulation and the informed consent process has been altered to reflect these changes.

The section titled "Use of Placebo" has elicited significant scholarly debate. The 1996 revision of the DoH was the first to mention the use of placebo and, through subsequent revisions, the Declaration has become more restrictive in the use of placebos.[22] This section begins by stating that, "The benefits, risks, burdens and effectiveness of a new intervention must be tested against those of the best proven intervention(s)." Taken out of context, it might be thought that this precludes the use of placebo. Following this initial statement, the DoH provides 2 situations in which it condones placebo experimentation:

- No proven intervention exists for the condition being studied.
- Placebo or no intervention can be used if it is necessary to conduct the study and evaluate the effectiveness and safety of the intervention being studied.

The Declaration further stipulates that a placebo intervention can be used only if these situations will not expose the subjects to additional risk. The ethical connotations of using a placebo in clinical trials are obvious to clinicians who have considered performing research on a new intervention. When a treatment exists that has proved its effectiveness and safety in treating a particular condition, especially if that condition produces great morbidity or death, allocating a patient to a placebo group seems unethical because the patient would be denied the more effective treatment. A less obvious consideration that makes restricting placebo use acceptable is that it can allow an investigator to embellish the success of a new treatment. For example, if a new treatment is compared with only the placebo, the researcher simply needs to show that it is better than the placebo, not how it compares to alternative, nonplacebo interventions. However, investigators who wish to show that their new treatments are superior can simply choose a nonplacebo control treatment that has questionable efficacy.[45]

The first situation in which placebo-controlled trials are condoned by the DoH is straightforward and without much controversy, provided no proven intervention exists. The second situation is not as clear and contradictory opinions exist. The Declaration states that placebo-control trials are ethical if "compelling and sound methodological reasons" support their use to "determine the efficacy or safety of an intervention." Some clinicians argue in favor of this exemption, explaining that certain conditions have an indeterminate response to placebo; therefore, placebo-controlled trials must be used to show efficacy.[38] With this in mind, it must be understood that just because a placebo-controlled trial may provide the most efficient way to answer an investigator's question, it may not be the most ethical. Others argue that using a 3-armed trial, which involves testing the new treatment against both a placebo and the best current treatment, can provide a more equitable process of using a placebo.[46] Critics of the Declaration's opinion regarding placebos continue to explain that using placebos when comparators exist always has consequences for patients who are not given useful treatments for controlling their symptoms or changing disease outcome.[20] Some experts argue that, in addition to conditions for which no proven treatment exists, the placebo restriction of the Declaration does not apply to studies of nondebilitating, short-term illnesses such as headaches and colds.[46] The issue lacks clarity as discussion commences regarding what constitutes a nondebilitating, short-term illness. That not withstanding, the use of placebo has played a significant role in musculoskeletal research. According to one author, the use of placebo instead of interferon-β or glatiramer during 10 investigations of new agents against multiple sclerosis resulted in relapses that may have been avoided if the more effective treatment had not been withheld.[47] Many interventional investigations in sports medicine continue to use placebo controls, such as platelet-rich plasma for ankle sprains,[48] rotator cuff tendinopathy,[49] and hamstring injuries.[50]

In summary, the use of placebo-controlled trials is a controversial topic and the DoH has attempted to restrict their use with the most ethically stringent guidelines in mind. Because of the complexity of this issue, more changes to this section can be expected in future revisions of the Declaration. It is no surprise that the last sentence of the section states that, "Extreme care must be taken to avoid abuse of this option." There may be temptations to expedite the acquisition of favorable results for a treatment by using a placebo, but the patient's welfare can never be compromised.

Paragraph 35 of the DoH states that, "Every research study involving human subjects must be registered in a publicly accessible database before recruitment of the first subject." In the current research environment, most investigators are not adhering to this guideline. In 2014, an article evaluating the registration of observational studies involving human subjects noted that an estimated 2% of 2 million completed or ongoing studies were registered.[51] Regardless of the numbers, this portion of the DoH is ahead of its time in terms of standardizing registration of observational human studies. The registration of prospective human trials is more common. Regardless of the type of study being performed (prospective or observational), the registration process helps to minimize the publication and reporting biases.[52] It is able to do this mainly because it makes it more difficult to withhold undesired results.[45]

Paragraph 36 addresses the issue of dissemination of research results. It explicitly states that "researchers, authors, sponsors, editors, and publishers" all have an ethical obligation to circulate research results, whether negative or inconclusive, that are complete and accurate. Research on publication bias against negative or inconclusive results in orthopedic literature has shown that this is more frequently a consequence of withholding submissions than of manuscript rejection.[45,53,54]

The final section, titled "Unproven Interventions in Clinical Practice," includes paragraph 37. It describes the use of unproven treatments in the hope of saving lives, to reestablish health, or to alleviate suffering. These unproven treatments should be implemented only "where proven interventions do not exist or other known interventions have been ineffective," and "after seeking expert advice, with informed consent from the patient or a legally authorized representative." After reading the first sentence of this paragraph, the reader might imagine lifesaving, heroic measures in the intensive care unit that have no relationship with sports medicine. However, sports medicine practitioners are focused on alleviating a specific type of suffering that requires constant innovation. This innovation can be a simple alteration of medications injected for early stages of knee osteoarthritis, or a slight variation in a particular surgical technique. In contrast, a new surgical procedure or technology could be developed. Regardless of the significance of the treatment advancement, orthopedic surgeons are ethically bound to monitor the results that it produces. This monitoring can be through simple audits of the treatment algorithms or the submission of a research protocol. Furthermore, after the information is gathered, "where appropriate" it should be made publicly available. This last statement of the DoH ethically binds orthopedic surgeons to be responsible researchers.[45]

SUMMARY

Significant changes have taken place over the past century regarding research ethics, allowing the establishment of numerous codes and guidelines. In this article, some of the most important documents contributing to these changes are mentioned. The DoH, which is the most cited text on international research ethics, is explored in detail. In contrast with the other guidelines discussed, the DoH is revised periodically, which makes it highly applicable to sports medicine, which is rapidly changing and innovative. As pioneering treatment options are developed, reliance on evidence-based medicine is critical. Furthermore, treating surgeons rely on research data that have been compiled and disseminated in an ethical and honest manner. This reliance serves to avoid compromising patient care. In conclusion, the necessity for conducting ethical research is paramount, and use of the DoH guidelines is essential for a safe and informed sports medicine practice.

REFERENCES

1. Dhai A. The research ethics evolution: from Nuremberg to Helsinki. S Afr Med J 2014;104:178–80.
2. Emanuel E, Crouch R, Arras J, et al. Ethical and regulatory aspects of clinical research: readings and commentary. Baltimore (MD): Johns Hopkins University Press; 2003.
3. Human subjects research. European Research Ethics Web site. 2012. Available at: http://www.ethicsweb.eu/ere/forskningmanniska.shtml. Accessed June 8, 2015.
4. Lacorte L. Good clinical practice 101: an introduction. US Food and Drug Administration Web site. Available at: http://www.fda.gov/downloads/Training/CDRHLearn/UCM176414.pdf. Accessed June 8, 2015.
5. The Nuremberg Code. US Department of Health & Human Services Web site. 2005. Available at: http://www.hhs.gov/ohrp/archive/nurcode.html. Accessed June 8, 2015.
6. WMA Declaration of Helsinki – ethical principles for medical research involving human subjects. World Medical Association Web site. 2013. Available at: http://www.wma.net/en/30publications/10policies/b3/index.html. Accessed June 13, 2015.
7. The Belmont Report. US Department of Health & Human Services Web site. 1979. Available at: http://www.hhs.gov/ohrp/humansubjects/guidance/belmont.html. Accessed June 13, 2015.
8. The Tuskegee Timeline. Centers for Disease Control and Prevention Web site. 2013. Available at: http://www.cdc.gov/tuskegee/timeline.htm. Accessed June 13, 2015.
9. Efficacy guidelines. International Council for Harmonisation Web site. 1996. Available at: http://www.ich.org/products/guidelines/efficacy/article/efficacy-guidelines.html. Accessed June 13, 2015.
10. ISO 14155:2011. International Organization for Standardization Web site. 2011. Available at: http://www.iso.org/iso/catalogue_detail?csnumber=45557. Accessed June 13, 2015.
11. Federal policy for protection of human subjects ('common rule'). US Department of Health & Human Services Web site. 1991. Available at: http://www.hhs.gov/ohrp/humansubjects/commonrule/index.html. Accessed June 13, 2015.
12. Parsa-Parsi R, Ellis R, Wiesing U. Fifty years at the forefront of ethical guidance: the World Medical Association Declaration of Helsinki. South Med J 2014;107(7):405–6.

13. Colledge F, Elger BS. Impossible, impractical, and non-identifiable? New criteria regarding consent for human tissue research in the Declaration of Helsinki. Biopreserv Biobank 2013;11(3):149–52.
14. Lie RK, Emanuel E, Grady C, et al. The standard of care debate: the Declaration of Helsinki versus the international consensus opinion. J Med Ethics 2004;30: 190–3.
15. Reider B. Happy (belated) anniversary, Helsinki. Am J Sports Med 2015;43(3): 539–41.
16. Shaw D, McMahon A. Ethicovigilance in clinical trials. Bioethics 2013;27(9): 508–13.
17. Wilson CB. An updated Declaration of Helsinki will provide more protection. Nat Med 2013;19(6):664.
18. Mutheswamy V. The new 2013 seventh version of the Declaration of Helsinki - more old wine in a new bottle. Indian J Med Ethics 2014;11(1):2–4.
19. Coursen JS. Review of "Fifty years at the forefront of ethical guidance: the World Medical Association Declaration of Helsinki" by Parsa-Parsa RW, Ellis R, Weising Y in South Med J 107:405–406, 2014. J Craniofac Surg 2015;26(1):308.
20. Parsa-Parsi R, Blackmer J, Ehni HJ, et al. Reconsidering the Declaration of Helsinki [letter]. Lancet 2013;382:1246–7.
21. Mehta S, Myers TG, Lonner JH, et al. The ethics of sham surgery in clinical orthopaedic research. J Bone Joint Surg Am 2007;89(7):1650–3.
22. Carlson RV, Boyd KM, Webb DJ. The revision of the Declaration of Helsinki: past, present and future. Br J Clin Pharmacol 2004;57(6):695–713.
23. Riis P. Perspectives on the fifth revision of the Declaration of Helsinki. J Am Med Assoc 2000;284(23):3045–6.
24. Chirba MA, Sweetapple B, Hannon CP, et al. FDA regulation of adult stem cell therapies as used in sports medicine. J Knee Surg 2015;28:55–62.
25. Vangsness CT, Farr J, Boyd J, et al. Adult human mesenchymal stem cells delivered via intra-articular injection to the knee following partial medial meniscectomy: a randomized, double-blind, controlled study. J Bone Joint Surg Am 2014;96(2):90–8.
26. Somerson JS, Bhandari M, Vaughan CT, et al. Lack of diversity in orthopaedic trials conducted in the United States. J Bone Joint Surg Am 2014;9(7):e56.1–6.
27. Puri KS, Suresh KR, Gogtay NJ, et al. Declaration of Helsinki, 2008: implications for stakeholders in research. J Postgrad Med 2009;55(2):131–4.
28. Otado J, Kwagyan J, Edwards D, et al. Culturally competent strategies for recruitment and retention of African American populations into clinical trials. Clin Transl Sci 2015;1–7. http://dx.doi.org/10.1111/cts.12285.
29. Coleman C, Lemmens T, Mehra T, et al. Research ethics committees: basic concepts for capacity-building. Geneva (Switzerland): World Health Organization; 2009. Available at: http://www.who.int/ethics/Ethics_basic_concepts_ENG.pdf.
30. Ross A, Athanassoulis N. The role of research ethics committees in making decisions about risk. HEC Forum 2014;26:203–24.
31. Sihvonen R, Paavola M, Malmivaara A, et al. Arthroscopic partial meniscectomy versus sham surgery for a degenerative meniscal tear. N Engl J Med 2013; 369(26):2515–24.
32. Sutherland AG, Cuthbertson BH, Campbell M. Sham surgery studies. Arthroscopy 2014;30(11):1389.
33. Lubowitz JH, Provencher MT, Rossi MJ. Could the New England Journal of Medicine be biased against arthroscopic knee surgery? Part 2. Arthrosc J Arthrosc Relat Surg 2014;30(6):654–5.

34. Freshwater MF, Garcia-Zalisnak DE, González-Ortiz NE. Failure of plastic surgical clinical trials to document compliance with international ethical guidelines: a systematic review. J Plast Reconstr Aesthet Surg 2013;66:3–8.
35. Murphy S, Nolan C, O'Rourke C, et al. The reporting of research ethics committee approval and informed consent in otolaryngology journals. Clin Otolaryngol 2015; 40:36–40.
36. Strech D, Metz C, Knüppel H. Do editorial policies support ethical research? A thematic text analysis of author instructions in psychiatry journals. PLoS One 2014;9(6):1–5.
37. Belhekar MN, Bhalerao SS, Munshi RP. Ethics reporting practices in clinical research publications: a review of four Indian journals. Perspect Clin Res 2014; 5(3):129–33.
38. Millum J, Wendler D, Emanuel EJ. The 50th anniversary of the Declaration of Helsinki: progress but many remaining challenges. JAMA 2013;310(20):2143–4.
39. Cvetanovich GL, Fillingham YA, Harris JD, et al. Publication and level of evidence trends in the American Journal of Sports Medicine from 1996 to 2011. Am J Sports Med 2015;43(1):220–5.
40. Macklin R. Revising the Declaration of Helsinki: a work in progress. Indian J Med Ethics 2012;9(4):224–6.
41. Wolinsky H. The battle of Helsinki: Two troublesome paragraphs in the Declaration of Helsinki are causing a furore over medical research ethics. EMBO Rep 2006;7(7):670–2.
42. Palacios R. Post-trial access and the new version of the Declaration of Helsinki. Colomb Med 2013;44(4):206–7.
43. Wilson JF. Health insurance portability and accountability act privacy rule causes ongoing concerns among clinicians and researchers. Ann Intern Med 2006; 145(4):313–6.
44. Armstrong D, Kline-Rogers E, Jani SM, et al. Potential impact of the HIPAA privacy rule on data collection in a registry of patients with acute coronary syndrome. Arch Intern Med 2005;165:1125–9.
45. Reider B. Helsinki redux. Am J Sports Med 2015;43(4):791–3.
46. Vastag B. Helsinki discord? A controversial declaration. J Am Med Assoc 2000; 284(23):2983–6.
47. Garattini S, Bertelé V, Banzi R. Placebo? No thanks, it might be bad for me! Eur J Clin Pharmacol 2013;69:711–4.
48. Rowden A, Dominici P, D'Orazio J, et al. Double-blind, randomized, placebo-controlled study evaluating the use of platelet-rich plasma therapy (PRP) for acute ankle sprains in the emergency department. J Emerg Med 2015;49(4): 546–51.
49. Kesikburun S, Tan AK, Yilmaz B, et al. Platelet-rich plasma injections in the treatment of chronic rotator cuff tendinopathy: a randomized controlled trial with 1-year follow-up. Am J Sports Med 2013;41(11):2609–16.
50. Reurink G, Goudswaard GJ, Moen MH, et al. Rationale, secondary outcome scores and 1-year follow-up of a randomised trial of platelet-rich plasma injections in acute hamstring muscle injury: the Dutch Hamstring Injection Therapy Study. Br J Sports Med 2015;49(18):1206–12.
51. Dal-Ré R, Delgado M, Bolumar F. El registro de los estudios observacionales: es el momento de cumplir el requerimiento de la Declaración de Helsinki. Gac Sanit 2015;29(3):228–31.
52. Williams RJ, Tse T, Harlan WR, et al. Registration of observational studies: is it time? Can Med Assoc J 2010;182(15):1638–42.

53. Okike K, Kocher MS, Mehlman CT, et al. Publication bias in orthopaedic research: an analysis of scientific factors associated with publication in the Journal of Bone and Joint Surgery (American Volume). J Bone Joint Surg Am 2008;90(3):595–601.
54. Sprague S, Bhandari M, Devereaux PJ, et al. Barriers to full-text publication following presentation of abstracts at annual orthopaedic meetings. J Bone Joint Surg Am 2003;85(1):158–63.

Index

Note: Page numbers of article titles are in **boldface** type.

Clin Sports Med 35 (2016) 315–320
http://dx.doi.org/10.1016/S0278-5919(15)00146-5
0278-5919/16/$ – see front matter © 2016 Elsevier Inc. All rights reserved.

sportsmed.theclinics.com

Moving?

Make sure your subscription moves with you!

To notify us of your new address, find your **Clinics Account Number** (located on your mailing label above your name), and contact customer service at:

Email: journalscustomerservice-usa@elsevier.com

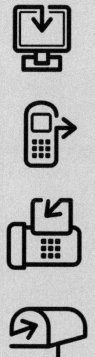

800-654-2452 (subscribers in the U.S. & Canada)
314-447-8871 (subscribers outside of the U.S. & Canada)

Fax number: 314-447-8029

Elsevier Health Sciences Division
Subscription Customer Service
3251 Riverport Lane
Maryland Heights, MO 63043

*To ensure uninterrupted delivery of your subscription, please notify us at least 4 weeks in advance of move.

Printed and bound by CPI Group (UK) Ltd, Croydon, CR0 4YY

08/05/2025

01864681-0001